MSAI
$4.95

In recent years American women have been attacked as frigid, castrating, and unfeeling. Beneath the veneer of attractive housewife, loving mother, and successful writer, the author of MY SELF AND I at first appears to be very much such a person. But during the 23 psychotherapeutic treatments she describes so dramatically, we witness the complete emotional regeneration of a modern woman.

Thanks to Constance A. Newland's unsparing honesty and rare bravery, here is the exciting and literally fantastic account of the unconscious forces which block personal fulfillment. Under psychiatry's new mind-loosening drug lysergic acid diethylamide-25, the powerful psychochemical that induces hallucinations, Mrs. Newland penetrates behind the paralyzing fear and the murderous rages that we all harbor within us. Her minute-by-minute journal of this struggle presents the reader with an unprecedented firsthand account of the still-uncharted regions of the unconscious: *"I traveled deep into the buried regions of the mind. I discovered that in addition to being, consciously, a loving mother and a respectable citizen, I was, unconsciously, a murderess, a pervert, a cannibal, a sadist, and a masochist. But in the wake of these dread discoveries I lost my fears . . . and I achieved complete sexual fulfillment."*

Praised by psychiatrists for its value as the first case history by an LSD patient, MY SELF AND I is even more important as a human document dealing with life's major themes, love and hate. Other writers have cited fear and anxiety as the principal obstacles to emotional fulfillment, but Mrs. Newland has had the courage to admit that the *real* destructive force—deeper and more powerful than fear—is suppressed rage and hatred.

Third Impression   0562

MY SELF AND I

My Self and I

CONSTANCE A. NEWLAND

FOREWORD BY *Dr. Harold Greenwald*

INTRODUCTION BY *Dr. R. A. Sandison*

Coward-McCann, Inc. New York

Contents

FOREWORD BY DR. HAROLD GREENWALD, 7

INTRODUCTION BY DR. R. A. SANDISON, 11

I. THE WAY TO LSD

    1. Myself, 19
    2. The Unconscious, 23
    3. The Drug, 37

II. THE CASE HISTORY

    4. The Closed-Up Clam, 55
    5. The Resistance, 65
    6. The Battle of the Sphincters, 73
    7. The Screams, 77
    8. The Purple Screw, 81
    9. The Cedar Chest, 93
   10. Collapse, 102
   11. The Purplish Poisonous Peapod, 104
   12. Venus Risen from the Sea, 127
   13. The Slim Black Nozzle, 136
   14. Celle Qui Fût la Belle Heaulmière, 150
   15. The "Ticking," 157
   16. The Return of the Full Bladder, 178
   17. The Bitten-Off Nipple, 193

III. MY SELF AND I

18. The Scared Spermatozoon, 207
19. The Malevolent Maggot, 214
20. The Gorgon, 217
21. The God of Wrath, 222
22. Empty Ecstasy, 225
23. The Grand Canyon, 228
24. The Riddle of the Sphinx, 229
25. My Self and I, 231

EPILOGUE

Now, 239

APPENDICES

APPENDIX A: LSD-25, 247

APPENDIX B: REALITY VERSUS PSYCHIC REALITY, 264

APPENDIX C: DISPLACEMENT, 268

APPENDIX D: PUNS AND WORD PLAY, 272

APPENDIX E: THE TRAUMA, 276

NOTES AND REFERENCES, 281

BIBLIOGRAPHY, 285

Foreword

By HAROLD GREENWALD, PH.D.

TELEVISION pundits, magazine savants and newspaper misogynists have been attacking the overwhelming majority of American women as being frigid, castrating and unfeeling.

At the start of the psychotherapeutic experience she describes so dramatically, the author of this book appears to be very much such a woman. She seems to be the very model of the frozen, ruthlessly efficient American career woman.

Now, thanks to her honesty, we have an exciting and literally fantastic account of the unconscious determinants of her attitudes and behavior. Unsparingly and with rare bravery, she discloses the fear and anxiety which was hidden behind what seemed like impregnable resistance. Thanks to the daring skill of her therapist, but even more to her own bravery in facing her rage, her fear, and her LSD-induced psychotic-like fantasies, she penetrated behind them to win understanding for herself and to present us with an unprecedented firsthand account of the still uncharted regions that we too glibly refer to as the unconscious.

Usually the nether regions of our own private infernos have been described for us by the comparatively cold scientific objectivity of the psychoanalyst. In this book, one of a small but growing list, we are, instead, given a first-person human account of one who has been there. Unflinchingly, the author depicts for us the paralyzing fear and the murderous rages that we all harbor within us and which threaten constantly to break through the thin veneer that civilization has created. At this particular moment of history these forces of fear and rage threaten not only to destroy our individual veneer, but life itself.

It will perhaps be easy for many readers of this book to close their eyes to the searing light Miss Newland casts on her own personal inferno by dismissing her as "disturbed" or "crazy"

7

or "sick"; if so, it will be only because they are not ready to bring her kind of courage to the task of self-inspection. To me it seems quite clear that most people meeting her even before her experience in self-discovery would probably have considered her well balanced, adjusted, or emotionally mature. That is another of the unique contributions of this book. It is not the account of the struggle to sanity of a raging schizophrenic or even the return to functioning of a severely crippled neurotic, but the further advance to self-realization of an already efficient, able member of society.

Dr. R. A. Sandison, the prominent authority on the use of LSD, in his Preface has described this book as being about the use of LSD in psychotherapy. It is that, of course, and such an excellent exposition of the use of the drug that I am even now engaged with a medical colleague in exploring this avenue of approach. My decision was based almost entirely on reading this book in manuscript and some of the literature to which it refers. In the constant battle we wage against human suffering, none of us in the therapeutic profession can afford to neglect exploring any new pathway that is offered to us, particularly one which gives hope of reaching the so-called "untreatable" patient, or the more numerous ones where we have had to settle for very modest goals indeed.

One of the impressive aspects of this book is that unlike many others who have written about relatively new forms of treatment, whether it is a new diet or a regimen of exercises, Miss Newland is not a special pleader. She makes no grandiose claims for LSD therapy as the one and only way to help, and carefully refrains from recommending it. Many of the disappointments with other forms of treatment have arisen from the too enthusiastic claims of some of its devotees.

However, valuable as the description of this new therapy may be, its real contributions lie in more important directions. First of all, this book is a literary document dealing in emotional, not clinical, terms with the major themes of life, love and hate. With excitement, we share the author's oft-terrifying, sometimes amusing journey of self-discovery. Apparently inexplicable nightmares and weird fantasies are explored to help us understand their meaning more clearly. In the course of this journey several other themes are illuminated.

Again, as I see in my daily practice, the depths of human negativity and resistance are plumbed. It is here that the skills of Dr. M. are most evident. His sensitive handling of the resistance, knowing when to bend with it and when to challenge it, is to my mind at least as valuable as the drug LSD in the successful outcome.

The whole baffling problem of frigidity in the liberally educated modern woman, who consciously has accepted her right to sexual pleasure but whose unconscious holds her frozen in the grip of fulfillment-destroying terrors and rages, is illuminated in a perceptive manner. Not the conscious anti-sexual teachings but the whole fabric of early relationships and experiences is exposed as the pleasure-destroying element. The intimate explorations of a woman's sexual life by a woman is practically unique in literature. Most such accounts have been written from the point of view of the man. Many accounts have been perceptive and intuitive but none to my knowledge has been able to tell us so much about the inner experiences of a woman's sexual response.

The chief concentration of most previous self-explorations in therapy has been on the fears of the individual. Lucy Freeman called her trail-blazing description of her analysis *Fight Against Fear*. Fear to most of us is a more readily admissible emotion than rage and hatred. For the same reason suppressed and unacceptable rage and hatred are more often responsible for our desperate efforts to avoid exposing our inner selves to us and to others. Miss Newland in her book has permitted us to see the rage and hatred she had previously not been able to admit existed.

But perhaps most important of all is that by telling us so much about one individual we learn a great deal about ourselves and thereby all humanity. Miss Newland's courage in facing the dark recesses of her own psyche should help us match her bravery in facing these same dark recesses in ourselves.

Introduction

By R. A. Sandison, B.Sc., M.B., D.P.M.

This is a book about the use of the drug LSD in psychotherapy. It is the first complete case history describing this treatment to be published, and it is significant that the author is not a therapist but a patient. Fortunately she is a gifted and imaginative woman whose account of her experiences during the LSD sessions carries the reader swiftly on through a series of psychological discoveries to a climax of unity and awareness of self.

LSD or lysergic acid diethylamide is one of a group of drugs usually called "hallucinogenic," a term which describes their power to produce so-called hallucinations in volunteer subjects. These random images become transformed into vivid fantasies when LSD is used in therapy and the drugs are thus better named "psycholytic" or "mind-loosening." These fantasies, developed by the patient under the careful direction of the therapist, bring into consciousness truths long hidden in the unconscious by fear, prejudice, and psychological resistance. This resistance, to which the author refers many times, is usually created by a one-sided attitude toward the unconscious. Such an attitude is clearly demonstrated by the author's failure to derive any understanding or benefit from orthodox psychoanalysis and by the long battle against Freudian principles in the first half of the book.

The twentieth century has translated the universal sickness of mankind into new languages, those of Freud, Jung, and Adler, followed later by newer contemporary schools of psychotherapy among which may be mentioned group, interpersonal, transactional, and existential therapies. Nearly all contemporary psychotherapies owe something to the principles laid down between 1890 and 1940 by Freud and Jung. What had in earlier times been regarded as possession by evil, weakness of will, sin, or moral and religious failure came to be regarded as the autonomous activity of emotional complexes whose true content was hidden from the patient in the unconscious, but which nevertheless altered the mood, behavior, and even thinking of the individual. Thus psychoanalytic theory has apparently to a large extent absolved man from responsibility for his actions. Nevertheless, orthodox beliefs continue to create for the neurotic and the deviant a load of guilt which is ill deserved. Psychiatrists have applied the term sickness to disorders within the unconscious, thus identifying mental with physical sickness and reviving the revolution of the eighteenth and nineteenth centuries during which physical illness gradually ceased to be considered the result of sin.

The reader may ask at this point why human life is so afflicted by the operation of unconscious conflicts; and what sense there can be in the co-existence of two minds, one conscious and the other buried, yet constantly at war with each other. It is believed that man in his primitive state lived almost entirely at the unconscious level, just as young children and old men and women and a few primitive peoples do today. These people have little individual existence; they are at the mercy of sympathetic magic, superstitious belief, and folklore. Their behavior is determined by taboo and ritual rather than by individual choice. Consciousness implies rational and factual explanations developed in man as part of the process of individuation. By the end of the nineteenth century this process in Europe and America had reached a climax of overvaluation of the rational and undervaluation of the spiritual. Man was henceforward to be an ordered being, the old mythologies had been purged and purified and were most fitted to be read by children; dreams, in the words of Sir Arthur Mitchell, were "sane hallucinations," whilst the scientists were wondering whether they had not now come to the end of their discoveries. Endless peace appeared to be in sight now that man had realized the folly of war. Two world wars and the no less revolutionary but less dramatic revelations of Freud and Jung drew man's attention to the fact that the unconscious was still the real force to be reckoned with in human affairs. Jung, in particular, felt that man's psychological development was only partially complete, and foresaw the next stage of his progress as one in which the unconscious contents would be drawn out into and integrated into consciousness, a process which he likened to man's old problem of reconciling the opposite in the transmutation of base metals into gold and which he called individuation. Psychoanalysis therefore sees in the unconscious part of the mind all the original potential of man's existence, perpetuated in myth, legend, and folklore, but kept in check by the ordered activity of awareness lest society be disrupted. Unhappily, the very forces which have created the unconscious have also created neurosis which in the individual causes much personal suffering and in the mass of mankind is responsible for those periodical social and political upheavals which now have reached such a scale that all human existence is threatened.

The author of *My Self and I* demonstrates clearly how intensely we hang on to well-tried conscious beliefs. She came into LSD therapy having already had an orthodox Freudian analysis. Although she had a clear intellectual understanding of Freudian theory she resisted any unconscious explanation for her symptoms. This resistance persisted well on into LSD treatment, but, despite this, the peculiar power of LSD to present unconscious contents as psychic realities brought about cure in the face of lingering doubts as to the apparently preposterous nature of the hypotheses. It was as if the mechanism of the neurosis, once uncovered, brought about cure in the presence of a skeptical attitude.

Those who read the pages which follow may wonder what theories there are to explain the action of the mind-loosening drugs. It will be remembered that the mental development of the child recapitulates that of the race, and that the psychic life of the young child is dictated by primitive and unconscious values. Magical beliefs, ritual and obsessional behavior, and fantasies which in adults might be regarded as psychotic pass as normal in young children. Not only this, but the child's mental life is closely tied to the unconscious life of the parents, particularly the mother, so that in some cases mother and child may have the same dreams. As the child grows he develops an ego life, which is sufficiently advanced by the age of 3 or 4 for the child to cease to refer to himself in the third person and by the age of 8 or 9 for him to feel himself to be a separate individual. But a single ego, or conscious image of self, does not form. Many images of oneself develop during the course of growing up. As many of the images conflict with preceding ones they tend to supercede each other, the earlier ones becoming unconscious. Thus the seven (or perhaps it should be many more) ages of man march on.

Those who practice therapy with LSD believe that the drug results in a selective undoing of the ego functions, each process uncovering and bringing into consciousness earlier ego images. Psychologically traumatic incidents in childhood tend to create their own ego images. For example, the sudden loss of a loved parent at a tender age creates a feeling that the emotions of bereavement will always exist unchanged, until time and the development of defensive processes buries the image where it lives on in the unconscious. Just how LSD dissolves ego images is unknown, but it has been observed for some years that patients in therapy relive the feelings and thoughts of childhood; that they can accurately say during the treatment session how old they feel. Furthermore, these experiences have often been completely forgotten, but their genuineness can sometimes be checked as in the author's experience with Miss Leahy and the enema. We should note also how clearly these early experiences refer to bodily sensations. Mrs. Newland refers repeatedly to these and has thus added much to the evidence that body and psyche are closely linked. Patients under LSD sometimes tell us that they are falling apart, or that they are dissolving or disappearing. Water, the universal solvent, often appears to surround them and one regards these experiences as symbols of ego disintegration. This thinning out of ego control may last for some hours and it gives the patient and the therapist an opportunity of exploring the unconscious. Consciousness is not lost and keeps a watching brief on the affair, being able to report events afterwards. In fact the author concedes that "LSD grants the faculty easily and effortlessly, to most people." She modestly avoids saying, however, that the process of making use of the faculty by the drug is a process of hard work and effort. Happily, it is not so demanding of time as psychoanalysis and in many cases the results are more rewarding.

Freud not only gave us a theory, he also gave us a method of treatment. The theory has proved to be the most adequate, the tools of treatment the least adequate. Free association and the interpretation of dreams are often insufficient to create psychic reality. The material presented in this book gives the clearest possible support for Freudian theory, and LSD therapists all over the world watch with fascination as the old truths which Freud enunciated come rolling out of the most unsophisticated patients. Jung gave us the method of active fantasy which the author has used with great effect during her treatment sessions. One should here comment on the sound principles of therapy which were used—encouraging the patient to live out the fantasies, to follow the LSD experience, and not to make suggestions nor to advise her. One is grateful that the circumstances of the therapy dispose of any idea, so often put forward, that the success of LSD therapy lies in suggesting psychoanalytic theories to the patient while she is in a suggestible state under the drug. In many passages in this book we have the clearest demonstration that the unconscious, left to itself, rejects suggestions it cannot use. It is our conscious minds that absorb suggestion.

Freud showed us that the mechanism of the unconscious is by word association, pun, wit, and humor. He also tells us that the unconscious is equally at home with the funny as it is with the squalid and the perverted. These principles are beautifully demonstrated in the text: the Purple Screw, the Purplish Peapod, the Amethyst Necklace, Inviolate or In Violet, the Blue Father and the Red Baby, the Fur Thing; all these share the same nest with jealousy, murder, castration, incest, and rape. Yet this is not childish fun or a horror comic, but the serious age-old mind material which lies within us all. Particularly impressive is the dream of the "barbarian shock troops" which appeared utterly incomprehensible to the patient on waking, yet whose meaning became crystal clear once LSD had been taken. This, incidentally, is the only time that LSD appears as a "bad object," which may relieve the misgivings which some Jungian therapists may have about the use of a drug to advance psychotherapy.

Later on, the narrative leads us beyond the frontiers of the personal unconscious into the impersonal or collective, that area of mind common to us all in which lie the archetypes which are the result of all man's past experience of special psychic images. Glimpses of the serpent and sphinx, the Old Wise Man and the God of Wrath, All-man and All-woman are sufficiently intriguing for us to hope that one day the author will give us another book devoted to the process of individuation, a process which she foreshadows in her finally reported experience of David and the Woman. In this experience, the title of the book is explained, that of the relationship between the totality of the psychic self and the "I," formerly considered all important, but now transformed.

In review, this book bears the stamp of authenticity, and its pages reveal situations and material which are very familiar to psycholytic therapists. It must be remembered that we are still far from perfecting this treatment, and that if its many dangers are to be avoided it must be carried out in a hospital or clinic environment by skilled therapists.

The pages which follow are a most valuable contribution to world literature and will be equally interesting to the therapists in many countries who have pioneered this treatment during the past eight years, and also to a great diversity of professional and lay people.

All will learn something more about the way in which advancing knowledge is helping to solve the problems of individuals today.

I

The Way to LSD

THE MIRACLE OF I

There is nothing in the world
More marvelous
Than I.
The living, breathing miracle of I.

The I of him;
The I of thee;
And, too, the I of me.

Anon

I.

Myself

"In her dark womb we did not know our mother's face; from the prison of her flesh have we come into the unspeakable and incommunicable prison of this earth. Which of us has known his brother? Which of us has looked into his father's heart? Which of us is not, forever, a stranger and alone?" [1]

One is tempted to add: Which of us has known himself? "Know thyself," the ancient maxim advises, but regrettably it does not tell us how. A man can learn to know his physical characteristics easily. With a little more difficulty he can learn his mental and even his emotional nature. It is a far more difficult thing to learn to *control* one's behavior, whether mental, physical, or emotional. It seems that self-knowledge is an ever deepening process. One begins with surface characteristics and then, layer by layer, seeks to penetrate to the innermost core of identity. But: how?

Quite by chance, three years ago, I found a way. And yet three years ago I thought that I knew myself rather well: a widow of respectable age and weight and height, in excellent health, who loved and cared for her children by pursuing a career as a writer. All in all, mine seemed a busy life and a pleasant one—though not carefree. I had a normal assortment of problems. For example, despite good health, I was troubled

19

by a chronic insomnia; and if I worked too long at my desk I suffered painful tensions in my arms; and occasionally I would be embarrassed by a silly sort of tic—my neck and throat would produce an odd clicking sound which would last for a minute or two and then disappear as suddenly as it had come. And there were other quirks. I could not fall asleep at night with a clock ticking in my bedroom; I had an abiding dread of dentists and would panic in a dentist's chair; and I would sometimes sink into moods of depression.

And more important than any of these: I had always been sexually frigid.

But none of these problems did I consider serious. Not even the frigidity, for I enjoyed the act of love immensely, even without fulfillment. Besides, I had been psychoanalyzed and had come to the realization that since I could not overcome the handicap, I could accept it gracefully. And finally I knew from friends (and from Dr. Kinsey, who reports that approximately one third of American women suffer similarly[2]) that frigidity among women is almost as prevalent as the common cold—and just about as incurable.

Three years ago, then, I thought myself a relatively healthy and happy woman. Some years before that time, I emphatically did not. Two days after our second child was born, my husband had died. I felt shipwrecked and sank into a profound sea of depression out of which, somehow, gradually, I was guided to shore, where I was able to build a new home for my children and a new career with which to provide for them. I became a commercial writer, successful to the point that I was being offered more assignments than I could manage. Meanwhile, new circles of friends appeared who entertained me, and whom in return I entertained in my comfortable home. All quite charming.

If I were to have named one lack in my life at that time I would have answered promptly: a man. It was not my children nor my work around which my life revolved, but rather the search for someone who would complete me. I even felt that

I had found such a man—only to face the impasse that he did not return my love, at least not enough to marry me. To compound this difficulty, he lived far away, so that we saw each other rarely. The few times we did see each other were very pleasurable, and very painful. For we would inevitably become involved in a quarrel which untied whatever unity we had found. I knew the romance was untenable, and that I must find someone else. Yet I clung to the romance because it helped fill the void within me. All the while I clung to it, I kept indulging in rounds of parties, laughter, and casual friends, and kept writing the slick fiction for which I was getting very well paid. I also cared for my children, as a good mother should. I always made sure that they were well-clothed and well-fed and well-schooled. True, I did not spend much time with the children but as I could logically argue with myself, and did, I had too much work to do. Besides, I further argued, my younger child was too small to need much of my time. Even as I argued, I recognized that last as an empty excuse. The birth of my daughter had become so interwoven in my mind with the death of my husband that it was painful for me to see or be with her during the whole first year of her life. I understood that this was wrong and irrational of me. Of course her life had not been made possible through the loss of my husband's life. I determined to overcome my unreasonable antipathy and did to the point that I was able to play and laugh with my daughter, peripheral as those actions may have been.

Altogether, then, I felt that I had learned to cope with the major problems of my life and was pleased with myself that I had. Furthermore, I reasoned since I functioned so well on a conscious level, there was no need to bother with those unconscious processes of mind which had concerned me during psychoanalysis. That unconscious mind had always seemed unreal to me, anyhow. Now it seemed irrelevant, for I was after all living the high life professionally and socially, besides being a loving mother and a law-abiding citizen.

It was at just that juncture that I volunteered for an experiment in psychotherapy. Feeling so well as I have professed, why did I submit myself to the experiment? I did not know the answer to that question then. It was only after my explorations were done that I found an answer: I had been propelled by a strong unconscious motive. But that answer would not have satisfied me when I volunteered for the experiment because, as I have indicated, at that time I did not accept the unconscious mind except as an interesting abstraction of small pragmatic value.

During the course of therapy I traveled deep into those remarkable regions of the mind and came upon a series of illuminations. I found that in addition to being, consciously, a loving mother and respectable citizen, I was also, unconsciously, a murderess, a pervert, a cannibal, a sadist, and a masochist. In the wake of these dreadful discoveries, I lost my fear of dentists, the clicking in my neck and throat, the arm tensions, and my dislike of clocks ticking in the bedroom. I also achieved transcendent sexual fulfillment.

Beyond these things, experiences nonpareil. I felt that I became—literally—a closed-up clam at the bottom of the sea, the music of a violin, Botticelli's "Birth of Venus," an evil fur thing, a scared sperm; and in one magnificent episode, it was as if I had become the very Energy that exists before it is translated into Matter.

These unsurpassed events occurred in that far reach of the mind, the unconscious, which had previously seemed an inaccessible myth. Now it became reality, amazingly accessible, simply through the taking of a drug.

This book strives to render an account of those experiences. It is, in effect, a case history—my own. It is also, perhaps more importantly, a description of an adventure in the unconscious human mind, as revealed through a chemical agency.

Before offering that description, I should discuss briefly the nature of the unconscious, according to authorities, and the nature of the drug, lysergic acid-diethylamide-25, abbreviated in the laboratory, happily, into the three letters: LSD.

2.

The Unconscious

THE idea of an unconscious mind is an absurdity. *Mind* implies a state of awareness, and *unconscious* implies a state of unawareness. How then can there be an awareness which is not aware?

This is an argument which has many adherents. In fact, probably the majority of people today do not believe in an unconscious mind. Three years ago, I did not. Despite a psychoanalysis which went on for four years, fifty weeks a year, five days a week, fifty minutes a day. During most of those minutes I talked (and talked and talked) about my problems. Sometimes I cried about them. Occasionally, between talking and crying, I listened and learned a few postulates about the unconscious mind.

One of the things I learned was that the "royal road" to the unconscious lay in the interpretation of dreams. Obediently I would report a dream at the beginning of a session and then would give my associations to the dream—a process which would sometimes extend beyond the hour into the next day's hour, and the next, and the next, before the ever widening chain of free associations which would appear with each facet of the dream had been exhausted.

Eventually I grew to resent the procedure, for it took an inordinate amount of time, and money, to achieve a negligible result in terms of therapy, or even insight into my problems.

As a result I was not at all convinced that the "royal road" led anywhere of any value. Nor did the other roads to the unconscious, like free association or slips of the tongue.

En route, naturally, I learned the terminology: the Oedipus complex, and latent homosexuality, and penis envy, and castration anxiety, and sibling rivalry, and so on and on. But I never came to grips with those concepts except intellectually. Hence, unconvincingly.

In the years after analysis, whatever validity the unconscious mind had had for me faded rapidly, while the phrases I had learned in the doctor's office became more and more prominent in plays, paperbacks, cocktail conversations, and even at PTA meetings.

This is not to say, of course, that such themes are unique to our society. Not at all. The Bible has a goodly share of tales involving incest, sodomy, sibling rivalry, mutilation, and murder. So has the Greek drama. So has Shakespeare. (It is surprising, incidentally, that so little attention is being given to Shakespeare's *Titus Andronicus,* a fund of perverse sex and mutilation, ending in an orgy of cannibalism that pales the plays of Tennessee Williams.) Emphatically, such themes are not new. Nor is such behavior.

However, it is a tragic fact that the first half of the twentieth century has unleashed the most massive depravities in recorded history. One has only to remember the "scientific" torture of human beings by the Nazis and the living skeletons found in their concentration camps, the deliberate mass starvation of peasants after the Russian revolution, the holocaust at Hiroshima, to realize that sadism and mutilation and aggression and destruction are not rare phenomena found only in abnormal or psychotic individuals.

Research into the causes and prevention of such behavior—which conceivably can annihilate mankind—is imperative. Some of this research has traveled in search of the causes and cures into the realm of the unconscious. And there the research has floundered—to the point of ridicule.

It would be a most unusual day on the American scene to find no derisive mention of "head-shrinkers" or "kooks." A head-shrinker, as any clear-thinking American knows, is not an African tribesman but a doctor concerned with mental health. And a kook is not an inmate of a mental hospital but an individual with some oddity of behavior. These oddities can range from unreasonable fears (of airplanes or spiders or pussy willows or swimming pools); to equally unreasonable desires (for the wild speed of a hot rod, for sex or alcoholic or eating orgies); to bizarre tastes (shaving one's head, saving daily newspapers, sleeping at the foot of the bed); to physical complaints which have no organic basis (lower back pain, stuttering, hysterical blindness or deafness or paralysis); all the way through to genuine illness (stomach ulcers, asthma, migraine headaches). A person suffering some such disability is regarded either as a figure of fun (the beatnik), or as a victim of fate to be treated with compassion because he is "sick." If a man is sick because he drinks too much before or instead of dinner, it may be explained on pseudo-psychiatric grounds that he was weaned too soon as a baby and never did satisfy his oral need for the bottle. If a woman is sick because she faints at the sight or mention of spiders, it may be similarly explained that she suffered a trauma in her childhood like that of Little Miss Muffet who panicked when that spider sat down beside her.

Such "Freudian" interpretations are legion—and ludicrous. Consider, for example, the innumerable references in today's literature to the phallic symbol. Pencils and cigars and umbrellas and skyscrapers and canes and totem poles and daggers and dirigibles have been so described; so has Cleopatra's Needle; and so has the austere Washington Monument. Recently a night-club comedian was richly rewarded with laughter when he told of offering a cigarette to a girl who eyed him coldly and challenged: "Do you know what you're *really* offering me?"

Ridicule. Which, in a way, is understandable. After all, the idea of an unconscious mind is a relatively new one, and new ideas are often derided. People laughed at Copernicus and Columbus and Darwin and Van Gogh and the Wright brothers. They probably laughed when that first cave man grunted his discovery of starting a fire by rubbing two sticks together. They probably would have laughed at Einstein could they have understood him.

And why should they not have laughed??

Suppose Columbus had asked you, a practical businessman, to finance an expedition across the Atlantic Ocean in order to reach India, a country you knew lay in the opposite direction? Patently Columbus belonged to the lunatic fringe who believe the world is round. Anyone with eyes in his head could see that the world is flat. As for the Wright brothers? Pitiful, in a ridiculous way of course, trying year after year to lift a heavy machine into the air. Anyone with common sense knew that nothing heavier than air could rise. All you had to do to prove it, as Newton had done, was to watch an apple fall from a tree.

Freud? Just as ridiculous. Take that idea of his about dreams being wish fulfillment. As if anybody wishes to be chased by a tiger or gorilla, or to find himself sinking into quicksands, or to walk down the street with no clothes on! Or take another of his ideas, that people develop peculiar habits, or serious illnesses, because of something that happened when they were so little they can't even remember what that something was. In itself perhaps that idea might not be so bad, but Freud went on to describe some of the things people can't remember—and those things are downright disgusting. How could any decent human being say that a child at the age of three or four wants to have sexual relations with his father or mother?

Yes, these criticisms seem justifiable. Most people, like good scientists, want proof of what they are asked to believe. People did accept the fact that the world was round (in spite of the evidence of their eyes) when a man sailed due west, kept sailing west, and arrived right back where he started from, still sailing west. And they accepted the crackpot idea of a flying machine when they saw a machine flying. They even accepted the preposterous claim that the invisible can become visible when they saw events that were happening half way around the world appear on their television sets.

Undoubtedly they would accept the paradox of an unconscious mind, which operates within them without their awareness, if they could have the experience for themselves. Thus far very few people have had that experience. I have.

That statement is not a boast. It was not my skill nor talent nor knowledge that made possible my experience. By great good luck I was led into the depths of my unconscious mind, which I did not really believe existed. I arrived there with no more knowledge of its contents than I have already described. After therapy, and only then, I did considerable research into the nature of the unconscious in order to be better able to write this book. I discovered that some of my experiences in the unconscious—experiences I had thought too horrible or too fantastic to report—had already been abundantly described by several authorities. This was a startling corroboration after the fact.

"That's all very well," one might object, "but I still do not believe that there is an unconscious mind. I accept airplanes because I've flown in them. And I accept the visible invisible because I've watched the World Series in my living room. But I've never seen any evidence for an unconscious mind. What proof is there that it exists?"

A valid question. And reminiscent of the one asked by a woman buying a dog whistle, the kind pitched too high for human ears to hear. When the salesman brought her such a whistle, she looked puzzled and asked: "But how do I know that it works?" The enterprising salesman went out into the street with the whistle and the woman, found a dog, blew the whistle, and the dog came running. The whistle worked. Q.E.D.

In a similar way, scientists have shown that the unconscious "works" even though its workings are beyond our awareness.

One of the clearest demonstrations of its operation is to be found in the phenomenon of post-hypnotic suggestion. This phenomenon has been reproduced so many times in so many people that it can no longer be denied as a fact of human behavior. One documented example: Under hypnosis, a man was instructed that five minutes after being wakened he would go to a certain window in the room, pick up a flower pot from the window sill, take the flower pot to a sofa, and wrap a towel around it. He was also told that he would remember none of these instructions on waking. Shortly afterwards the subject was returned to consciousness. When asked what had happened to him while he had been hypnotized, the man replied that he did not know; he had simply felt as if he had been asleep.

Inconsequential talk followed, in which the man participated —until exactly five minutes after he had been wakened, he walked to the designated window, picked up the flower pot, carried it to a sofa and wrapped it around with a towel. When asked why he had done such strange things, the man looked bewildered and replied that he did not know; he just felt like it.

Some part of this man, clearly not his conscious mind, remembered and carried out a complex series of actions. What part of him was it? No region of the mind (or body) which performs this function has as yet been isolated—but wherever and whatever that region may prove to be, it has been given the name of the unconscious mind.

Another point of interest in this illustration: When the subject was urged, repeatedly, to explain his odd behavior, he gave several reasons for doing what he had done. First, he said that he had noticed the flower pot was in danger of falling from the window sill and had walked over to it to set it straight; on picking up the flower pot, he had realized it was cold because of the strong draft from the window; then he had decided to move it to the sofa and give it the warmth of a towel. Surely these were good and logical reasons to explain his behavior, but they were not the real reason, which he did not know.

How often in our daily lives do we give good and logical

reasons for a certain action, rather than the real reason—of which we may be totally unaware?

That is to ask: Why do you whistle a particular tune at a particular moment? Why do I, on impulse and in spite of my diet, decide to have an ice cream soda? Why do you, or I, feel so tired suddenly that we take an unaccustomed nap?

Most of us would probably answer: "I don't know, I just felt like it." An answer remarkably similar to that of the hypnotized subject when he was asked about his actions with the flower pot.

Furthermore, if I were urged (as the subject was urged) to give a specific reason for a specific behavior—why had I taken that ice cream soda?—I would probably offer a number of very good and convincing reasons: "Because I was thirsty. And it was hot. And besides, I needed some quick energy because I'd been dieting too strenuously. Anyhow, I was passing that shop where they make perfectly wonderful ice cream sodas, and I hadn't had one in ages."

Human beings are ingenious. We can invent an incredible number of credible reasons to explain why we do what we do—but often the real reason for a specific behavior remains concealed in the unconscious mind.

What else is concealed in the unconscious? It has been postulated by philosophers and scientists alike that every experience of the individual, from the moment of his birth, is imprinted in him for all of his life. Delboeuf wrote: "Every impression, even the most insignificant, leaves an unalterable trace [in the individual]." [1] Scholz claimed that "nothing we have once psychically possessed is ever entirely lost." [2] Pavlov, the Russian physiologist acclaimed for his discovery of the conditioned reflex, believed that all behavior evolves from the earliest, most primitive responses we make to our environment. "Different kinds of habits based on training, education, and discipline, are nothing but a long chain of conditioned reflexes." [3]

During the years that Pavlov worked in his laboratory, studying the behavior of dogs and other animals, Freud worked in his clinic, studying the behavior of his patients, and arrived at a similar conclusion: "The mortification suffered thirty years ago operates, after having gained access to the unconscious source of affect, during all those thirty years as though it were a recent experience. Nothing can be brought to an end in the unconscious: nothing is past or forgotten." [4]

These several statements were offered around the turn of the century. In more recent years, scientists working in different fields have found empirical evidence to support the hypothesis. A celebrated Canadian brain surgeon, Penfield, discovered that electrodes placed at certain points in the cerebral cortex will evoke long-buried incidents in the life of the patient whose brain is being so stimulated. It has also been proved, repeatedly, that under hypnosis a person will remember with astonishing accuracy such details as the clothes he was wearing or the food he ate on his fifth or fourth or even second birthday. And it has been found that certain drugs—including lysergic acid— will revive totally forgotten memories.

So the hypothesis has been offered by various authorities, with some evidence to support it, that no experience is lost to an individual. This concept has a number of startling implications. Consider this one: Imagine a charming lady with a little idiosyncrasy: She detests cats. She does not remember any incident, unpleasant or frightening, that happened to her which involved cats. She simply knows that she cannot bear to be near a cat; and if she is forced to be with one for any length of time, she develops a migraine headache. Why?

For answer, I should like briefly to describe an experiment performed by Watson and Reyner, in 1920.[5] Watson was impressed with Pavlov's work on conditioning emotional reactions in animals, and wanted to find out if emotions could be similarly conditioned in human beings. He was also particularly interested in how fear develops in a baby, and took as the subject for an experiment a nine-month-old boy, Albert, who was healthy, well-adjusted, and so little given to emotional outbursts that he was considered almost phlegmatic. Over a period of time, Watson tried to find some object which would evoke fear in Albert, using such things as masks, burning newspapers, a monkey, a dog, and a white rat. All of these left Albert quite undisturbed. Eventually Watson found one thing which frightened Albert so much that the child gasped, trembled, and began to cry. That thing was an unexpected, loud sound. On the basis of this finding (a finding known to almost every mother), Watson devised a remarkably simple experiment, and was able to condition Albert to be afraid of a white rat—of which Albert had previously not been afraid. All that Watson did was to present Albert with the white rat and, as Albert reached out and touched the creature, a loud and unexpected sound was made behind Albert's head. Immediately Albert jumped violently, fell forward, and began to whimper.

After a very few such experiences, Albert was shown the white rat, with no accompanying loud sound, and he immediately fell forward, cried, and tried to crawl away.

An astonishing aftermath of this experiment was that Albert's fear of the white rat spread to other objects which were furry, or white. For months afterward, if Albert were shown a dog, a rabbit, cotton wool, or a mask of Santa Claus with white whiskers, he would whimper and try to crawl away.

It is pleasant to report, by the way, that Watson offered various techniques to recondition Albert so that he would no longer be afraid of white rats or Santa Claus' whiskers.

But if no experience is ever lost to an individual, is it not conceivable that somewhere today there is a middle-aged man named Albert who becomes unaccountably uneasy whenever he sees Santa Claus? A middle-aged man would scarcely remember an episode that happened when he was a year old. And yet, according to current theory, both the episode and the emotion may have remained operative in him, unconsciously. So, too, it may have happened with our lady who, for no reason that she knows, detests cats. "The mortification suffered thirty years ago operates [unconsciously] . . . during all those . . . years as though it were a recent experience."

The unconscious might then be likened to an immense store-house which contains all of one's experiences, where one can find the real reason (rather than contrive good reasons) to explain one's actions: whether that action be an uncontrollable fear of white rats or spiders or ticking clocks; or an uncontrollable desire for liquor or sex—or an ice cream soda.

Accepting this concept of the unconscious, a strange idea presents itself. If an emotion experienced thirty years ago continues to operate *with its original intensity*, then it follows that the unconscious is a region in which *time is not a dimension*. As a matter of fact, Freud decided that "there is nothing corresponding to the idea of time, no recognition of the passage of time, and (a thing which is very remarkable and awaits adequate attention in philosophic thought) no alteration of mental processes by the passage of time." [6] Jung goes further and speaks of "the extraordinary timeless quality of the unconscious: everything has already happened and is yet unhappened." [7]

As we shall discover, this quality of timelessness is a phenomenon frequently experienced by people under the influence of LSD.

There remains only one more aspect of the unconscious to be examined, this one derived exclusively from Freud. Although Freud has grown out of fashion in recent years with some scientists, it cannot be denied that it was he who first constructed a working model of the unconscious mind. It can be denied that Freud discovered the unconscious. He did not—as he himself was quick to point out. He merely discovered its practical applications. "Probably but very few people have realized the momentous significance for science and life of the recognition of unconscious mental processes. It was not psychoanalysis, let us hasten to add, which took this first step. There are renowned names among the philosophers who may be cited as its predecessors. . . . Psychoanalysis has only this to its credit, that it has not affirmed these properties . . . on an *abstract* basis . . . but *it has demonstrated them in matters that touch every individual personally.*" [8]

Several other men in history, then, had come upon one or another wellspring of the unconscious, but it was Freud who deliberately drilled through the bedrock of consciousness to find its vast underground ocean, an ocean rather like the Atlantic Ocean of the Middle Ages: unexplored, uncharted, and thought to be inhabited by indescribable monsters waiting to destroy those who ventured too far into its depths. Freud ventured, explored—and came upon some of those indescribable monsters which he described in terms that have become as familiar in this our twentieth century as radar and television and supersonic satellites. I refer, of course, to those fulsome phrases sibling rivalry, Oedipus complex, castration anxiety, latent homosexuality, etc.

In his later years, Freud added a trio of terms to the list, a trio now well-worn but not well understood: the id, the ego, and the superego. Freud, by the way, did not use the words "ego" and "id," but rather the "I" and the "it." "You may feel dubious," he wrote, "over the choice of simple pronouns to designate our two psychical agencies or provinces, instead of high-sounding Greek names. *But in psychoanalysis we like to remain in touch with popular ways of thinking and we prefer to make use of everyday concepts* rather than to throw them away. That is no merit to us—we must proceed in this way, since our teaching must be understood by our patients who are often highly intelligent but not always highly educated." [9] At the end of this passage there is an asterisk and a translator's footnote: "In accordance with the usage adopted by psychoanalysts, these terms 'I' and 'It' have been replaced by Ego and Id throughout the remainder of this translation." *Sic transit gloria simplicitatis.*

Freud borrowed the word "It" (Id) from such colloquial expressions as "It bothers me very much" or "It made me so angry, I got drunk." This "It" which wells up and sometimes overwhelms us is primarily "an impulse to obtain satisfaction for instinctual needs." [10] In opposition to this impulsive "It," there is a rational "I" (Ego) which can usually control those impulses.

In a simile strangely evocative of Goya's "Young Woman on a Bucking Horse," Freud describes the Ego as "a man on horseback who has to hold in check the superior strength of the horse." [11] In Goya's etching the horse (the Id) is about to overthrow its rider (the Ego).

In addition to these two provinces of mind, Freud postulated a third province: the Superego, which can be roughly likened to one's conscience, one's code of morality. Like the Id, the Superego operates, for the most part, unconsciously. This statement, on first view, seems far-fetched. How can one's moral code be unconscious? Certainly one is very aware of what he believes to be right and wrong.

But just as the baby Albert developed a fear of white rats and cotton wool and Santa's whiskers, unconsciously, so does a baby develop, unconsciously, ideas of right and wrong. Even before he can talk, a baby learns that it is wrong to throw his bottle on the floor, wrong to wet his bed, wrong to smear the walls with dirty fingers; he also learns (one hopes) that it is right to go to the potty when necessary, right to eat certain things at certain times, right to obey his parents. From such simple processes, according to Pavlov, evolve the most complex behaviors of adult life, including a code of ethics to which one subscribes.

These then, the Id, Ego, and Superego, are the Big Three which coexist within each one of us. Often, "I want to" fights against "I must not," and the mediator in the conflict is one's rational, conscious Ego.

Most of us, most of the time, are able to resolve such conflicts. Occasionally, of course, "I want to" triumphs over "I must not" —and I indulge in that ice cream soda in spite of the diet. Conversely, "I must not" wins out, and I deny myself that long-planned vacation because it would be "wrong" to leave the children. But generally, the majority of men manage a working equilibrium.

Some do not. Probably we all know a man or woman who is propelled from one promiscuity to another, or who gets drunk too often, or who loses job after job because of an uncontrollable temper. These are the riders whose horses keep running away with them. Often these people will give ingeniously good reasons to explain how they were caught up in that last wild binge, or why they had to blow up at the boss, or why it was imperative to get that second divorce to make way for the third marriage. . . .

At the opposite pole are those people who are so fearful or who feel so guilty that they must constantly apologize for whatever they do. A friend once described to me the deathbed scene of his father, a meek and ineffectual man, whose last words to his family were: "Excuse me. . . ."

Either extreme can be disastrous. Joe, for example, is a heavy drinker—but he will explain, convincingly, why any specific drunken night was a necessity: "My mother-in-law was bugging me so much, I had to get crocked or I'd have slugged her." "I had such a rotten week at the office, I needed a few just to take my mind off my problems." "The kids were making such a racket, I had to get out of the house and blow off steam for a while."

But Joe may get drunk more and more often, until he loses a weekend or two—and then finds himself on Skid Row, an alcoholic.

Ellen, on the other hand, refuses to go out with the men who invite her, always offering excellent reasons why: "It wouldn't be right to leave mother alone when she isn't feeling well." "It would be wrong of me to go out tonight when I have so much studying to do." "But I can't go out with him! He isn't nice at all! You should see the way he looks at me. . . ." After a time Ellen may refuse to go out with anyone, ever, because she is afraid of—something. This vague fear may remain vague, or it may develop into a conviction that it is dangerous for her to leave the house because someone is planning to murder her

—by which time she is ready to be hospitalized. Somewhere along the way Joe may come to the rough realization that he can no longer stop drinking even though he wants to stop. And Ellen may find that she is so afraid of "something" that she is compelled to look under her bed several times each night before she can fall asleep.

Both Joe and Ellen may reach the difficult decision that they need help. But what kind of help? And where can they find it?

There is a wide variety of help offered today, ranging from Alcoholics Anonymous to tranquilizers to psychiatric interviews to Christian Science to hypnotherapy to electro-shock treatment to sleep cures to psychoanalysis to the laying on of hands—a list far from inclusive.

Some of these treatments do not attempt to find the real reasons for irrational behavior like that of Joe or Ellen. Rather they strive to release the fears and anxieties which are crippling the patient. Sometimes these treatments succeed and the patient is cured. Often he is not.

Psychotherapists Freudian and neo-Freudian believe it is important to find the real reasons for the fears and anxieties that, like the Hound of Heaven, relentlessly pursue the sufferer; and they have developed various techniques to discover those reasons. Sometimes such analytic therapy succeeds and the patient is cured. Often he is not. "You are perhaps aware that I have never been a therapeutic enthusiast," Freud wrote, in his *New Introductory Lectures.* "The proportion of recoveries which have been effected gives us ground neither for boasting nor for feeling ashamed. . . . I may say that I do not think our successes can compete with those of Lourdes. There are so many more people who believe in the miracles of the Blessed Virgin than in the existence of the unconscious. But if we disregard supernatural competition, we must compare psychoanalysis with other methods of psychotherapy. . . ." [12]

Recently another form of psychotherapy has been added to the list: drug therapy. One of the drugs which is now being studied as a possible therapeutic agent is lysergic acid.

3.

The Drug

ALDOUS HUXLEY'S brilliant work *Heaven and Hell* describes "the antipodes of the mind," a realm of supernal vision and imagery, beyond Time, visited rarely in history by some few great artists and mystics—but a realm to which the ordinary man can now be temporarily transported by the taking of a harmless chemical:

"The typical mescaline or lysergic acid experience begins with perceptions of colored, moving, living geometric forms. In time, pure geometry becomes concrete, and the visionary perceives, not patterns, but patterned things such as carpets, carving, mosaics. These give place to vast and complicated buildings, in the midst of landscapes, which change continuously, passing from richness to more intensely colored richness, from grandeur to deepening grandeur. Heroic figures, of the kind that Blake called 'The Seraphim,' may make their appearance, alone or in multitudes. Fabulous animals move across the scene. Everything is novel and amazing . . . [The visionary] is looking on at a new creation." [1]

It was here that I first happened on the words "lysergic acid." So enthralling were Mr. Huxley's descriptions of the "new creation" that I determined to have the experience myself—sometime. For several years that time did not present itself. Then quite by accident I learned of a research project in psychotherapy involving the use of lysergic acid. Psychotherapy seemed a province so far removed from the visionary experiences described by Mr. Huxley as to be absurd. But on an impulse (an impulse as unfathomable as the whistling of a particular tune at a particular time) I volunteered for the experiment.

In a preliminary talk with the doctor in charge, I was told that LSD was not habit-forming, that it was not harmful physically, and that its effects—if too overwhelming psychologically—could be swiftly curtailed by the administration of an antidote.

These bare facts, plus the fabulous reports of Mr. Huxley, made up the sum of my knowledge about lysergic acid when I began therapy. After therapy, again *only* after therapy, I did research into the nature and history of the drug from the moment its remarkable qualities were discovered, in 1943.[2]

LSD, along with several other drugs, has been classified as an hallucinogen because these drugs cause hallucinations.

But what is an hallucination? The dictionary offers as a psychological definition of hallucination "an auditory or visual sensation originating in the mind without external stimulation."[3] Most people tend to consider hallucinations as belonging to the fringes of human behavior. An alcoholic in the throes of delirium tremens will see hordes of attacking cockroaches or those notorious pink elephants; victims of prolonged thirst will see, far off in the desert, lakes of blue, blue water; psychotics of a certain kind will spend hours conversing with people who are invisible. Hallucinations such as these are certainly abnormal phenomena.

All the same, it is not an extravagance to say that everyone has hallucinations. Who has not, at one time or another, heard footsteps in the dark, footsteps which existed only in his imagination? Who among us has not seen a friend on the street and hurried to meet him only to be confronted with a stranger? Who among us has not dreamed a dream?

It is difficult at first to reconcile a dream with an hallucination—until one tries to define a dream. Attempting such a definition in *The Interpretation of Dreams,* Freud quoted from various authorities, all the way back to Aristotle. Out of these many quotations he distilled two facts concerning the nature of a dream: that a dream is made up preponderantly of visual images, and "without entering upon a discussion of the nature of hallucinations—a discussion familiar to every psychiatrist—we may say, with every well-informed authority, that the dream *hallucinates.*" [4]

Stop to consider: in a vivid dream, one flies in an airplane, or walks down the streets of his childhood, or talks with someone long since dead—and it is only *after* waking, usually, that one realizes those events were "auditory or visual sensations originating in the mind without external stimulation." Let us accept the opinion of "every well-informed authority" and grant that the dream is an hallucination. Usually dreams (or hallucinations) appear when one is asleep, which is to say when one's five senses are for the most part quiescent. Under LSD, however, hallucinations (or dreams) appear while one's five senses are actively functioning, *while one is awake*—a paradox. How can a person be awake and dreaming at the same time?

Such a state of double awareness (or split in the personality) would seem to belong, like hallucinations, to the sphere of abnormal phenomena. But, again like hallucinations, double identity is an experience which occurs almost universally. Who among us has not, at one time or another, daydreamed something to the effect that he is eloping with his ideal woman, or that he is the first astronaut to land on Mars, or that he is pitching a no-hit game in the World Series—*while at the same time* he hears, and obeys, the call to dinner? Under circumstances like these, a person operates on two levels of consciousness simultaneously, and effectively too.

So valuable for therapy did Jung find this state of double awareness that he tried to evoke it deliberately in his patients through a technique called "active imagination." "One concentrates one's attention on . . . a spontaneous visual impression and observes the changes taking place in it. . . . Long and often very dramatic series of fantasies ensue. . . . Once a visual series has become dramatic, it can easily pass over into the auditive or linguistic sphere and give rise to dialogues and the like. . . . [Such fantasies] differ from dreams only by reason of their better form, which comes from the fact that *the contents were perceived not by a dreaming* but by a waking consciousness." [5] Jung goes on to caution that this state of double identity is difficult to achieve, and that not many patients can develop the faculty. LSD grants the faculty easily, and effortlessly, to most people.

But why is the ability of being awake and dreaming at the same time considered valuable, therapeutically? Before answering this question, it is necessary to understand why dreams (or fantasies or hallucinations) are used again and again in psychotherapy. And they are so used, not only by Jungian and Freudian analysts, but by psychiatrists and psychologists and psychotherapists of almost every school.

One standard procedure in evaluating personality today is the administration of the Rorschach test. This consists of a series of cards, on each of which is printed an inkblot of ambiguous form, which the patient is asked to describe in detail. In other words, he is asked to fantasy or dream up images and stories out of the vague impressions which are presented to him. Other standard procedures include modeling in clay, acting out scenes with dolls or with other people, finger painting, and tests like the thematic apperception test. All of these devices attempt to discover, *through fantasy,* the dynamics of the patient's personality; to discover his underlying conflicts, or anxieties, or guilts—which frequently he is unable to define consciously.

As illustration on a simple level, let us explore the daydream of being the first astronaut to land on Mars. A man inclined to this fantasy would perhaps be a person who wants to get away from his humdrum existence, to explore and adventure, and to be acclaimed for his efforts not only by the world, but also, importantly, by himself. This fantasy, or daydream, could then be interpreted as a desire for adventure, and esteem.

But the majority of fantasies and dreams are not so simply constructed. How interpret this recurrent nightmare? Mr. X dreams that he is a child in school being taught by a teacher who looks exactly like the corner grocer. Suddenly the teacher transforms into a gorilla who pursues Mr. X, no longer a child but himself the man, through a swampy forest until he stumbles over a precipice and is plunging headlong toward an active volcano, screaming, screaming as he tumbles downward—only to wake up, terrified, in the middle of a scream.

Apart from Mr. X's very real terror, the events in the dream seem so unreal to him as to be absurd. Why should his teacher have been the corner grocer? And how, in an instant, could the grocer become a gorilla, and the boy a man? And what are the swampy forest lands that lead precipitately to an abyss?

Since the majority of dreams contain irrational elements like these, they were long dismissed as incomprehensible and meaningless phenomena—"the excreta of the mind." Freud, however, spent a great part of his life studying these "meaningless" phenomena, and came upon profound meanings, which could be revealed by asking the dreamer to say whatever came into his head about different aspects of the dream.

Let us use as an example one aspect of the nightmare just described: the teacher-grocer-gorilla. If Mr. X were to report whatever ideas or thoughts occurred to him about the schoolteacher in the dream, he might remember a specific incident concerning a specific teacher, which would relate somehow to the corner grocer, which in turn might relate to Mr. X's concept of a gorilla. Each of these three separate and seemingly disparate images, then, might become a *symbol* for one specific problem—whether a fear or a guilt or an anxiety or even a disguised wish.

Both Jung and Freud, moreover, noticed that certain images appeared again and again in the dreams of various patients. With remarkable consistency such images as daggers, caves, spiders, forests, guns, seagulls, kitchens, oceans, volcanoes, ships, gorillas, et cetera, would be reported in dreams and these images were discovered to have a meaning common to all the dreamers. In other words, dream imagery was discovered to be a kind of symbolic language.

I had learned this fact, intellectually, during psychoanalysis but, for whatever reason, I had not felt its emotional truth. But under LSD I found myself repeatedly in the midst of extraordinary imagery, such as a whirlwind, the labyrinths of Hades, a Black Mass, the cave of the Gorgon, monsters of Hieronymous Bosch (to mention only a few): and even as I saw these images, I sometimes recognized them for what they were meant to symbolize. At other times, I did not appreciate their significance until later. As a specific instance of the latter, on one occasion I saw a vague but terrifying image of what I could only describe (and with difficulty) as a purplish, and poisonous peapod. Meaningless image. However, in a later session that image reappeared spontaneously. By concentrating on it, and by pursuing the fantasies which evolved from it—a variation of Jung's "active imagination"—I arrived at long forgotten episodes which not only made clear the meaning of that symbol, but which helped me to understand and then to conquer my hitherto unconquerable frigidity.

This is one great value of the faculty granted by LSD: of being awake and dreaming at the same time. One part of the person is able to participate in the events of a dream, while a second part of him is able to interpret the meaning of the dream or fantasy.

Not only do images and symbols appear under LSD but also isolated and apparently meaningless words. Freud came upon this phenomenon early in his career, when he was using hypnosis as an adjunct to therapy. One of his hypnotic techniques was to ask the patient to close his eyes and to report what he saw when Freud placed his hand on the patient's forehead. Employing this technique with a woman patient suffering from obsessions and phobias, Freud wrote:

> When I asked the lady whether she had seen anything or had any recollection under the pressure of my hand she replied:

"Neither the one nor the other, but a word has suddenly oc-curred to me."

"A single word?"

"Yes, but it sounds too silly."

"Say it all the same."

"Concierge."

"Nothing else?"

Once more an isolated word shot through her mind:

"Nightgown."

I saw now that this was a new sort of method . . . and I brought out what seemed to be a meaningless series of words. Concierge. Nightgown. Bed. Town. Farm cart.

"What does all this mean?" I asked.

She reflected for a moment and the following thought oc-curred to her:

"It must be the story that has just come into my head. When I was ten years old—my next eldest sister was twelve. She went raving mad one night and had to be tied down and taken into town on a farm cart. I remember perfectly that it was the concierge who overpowered her and afterwards went with her to the asylum as well." [6]

Those isolated and meaningless words had led the patient into the storehouse of her unconscious mind, there to discover a long buried experience which was significant in the evolution of her illness.

Once, under the double awareness of LSD, the conscious part of me heard the other part of me mumble two words: "Cedar chest . . ." The words sounded silly. They were incomprehen-sible. I knew nothing of any cedar chest. Those words, spon-taneously spoken, were isolated from all conscious thought. Gradually, though, other isolated words, and then images, be-gan to float to the surface and to cluster around the words "cedar chest." Then, memories began to emerge, memories of totally forgotten incidents which helped me to understand, and then to resolve, another of my difficulties.

Here is one more benefit to be derived from being awake and dreaming at the same time. One can hear isolated words emerge from somewhere within him, words which he can pursue consciously, to arrive perhaps at new, sometimes staggering, insights.

There are still other therapeutic values to be derived from the dual identity granted by LSD; values which can also be found, frequently, under hypnosis and sodium pentathol (more rarely with psychoanalysis).

One of these is "abreaction," meaning that a patient can be induced to *relive* a forgotten, or repressed, experience with all of its original emotional intensity, emotion which has remained bottled up inside him without his knowledge. When that emotion is released, the patient is sometimes relieved of his particular symptom, whether that symptom be hysterical blindness, or paralysis, or asthma, or obsession.

Regarding this phenomenon as it appears under LSD therapy, Dr. Sandison and his colleagues report: "We have been greatly impressed by this surging up of repressed experiences which has caused some of the most intense abreaction we have ever seen." [7]

I can corroborate this statement. Although I had never experienced any kind of abreaction before—and indeed did not believe that I was capable of doing so—under LSD I relived the strongest, most intense emotional experiences conceivable. In one session, suddenly and without warning, my arms propelled themselves across my chest and remained there as if they had been pinned into a strait jacket. I screamed and sweated and struggled to release them, panic growing in me all the while, but my arms lay as if paralyzed, and I could not move them. Actually, I was reliving an episode which had occurred when I was exactly two and a half years old, which I had totally forgotten. However, the experience had remained—along with the feelings of helplessness and terror it had engendered—for all the years between, without my knowledge. By reliving that experience, and by releasing the emotions it had created in me, I was subsequently relieved of the tensions in my arms which had plagued me chronically for several years as an adult.

In connection with this particular abreaction, an amazing thing happened. As my arms lay paralyzed across my chest, I felt that my body was dwindling in size, smaller and smaller, until I felt that I had become a baby. All the while I could hear and understand what the doctor was saying, but I could not answer him because, as a baby, I knew no words. When at length I was able to talk, it was with the limited vocabulary and lisping voice of a very small child. It was exactly as if, with one part of me, I had become a baby.

This phenomenon is called "age regression," and occurs frequently under hypnosis. A skilled hypnotist can regress a good subject back to his fifth, fourth, or even second year; and the subject will speak, move and behave like the five-year-old or two-year-old he has temporarily become. What is more, the subject will relive episodes out of those years in the most minute detail—detail which it has been possible, in some cases, to verify.

As we have seen, both age regression and abreaction occur in therapies other than LSD. But again there is the major advantage of LSD's dual awareness. One part of me, in the experience just described, had become a two-year-old baby, living through an extremely painful event in which my arms had been tied down so that I could not move them—but at the very same time I was also myself, a mature woman, observing what was happening, and able to correlate the excruciating arm tensions I was suffering in reliving that episode, to the chronic arm tensions I had been suffering for several years.

That particular symptom disappeared within a few weeks. It is important to realize that the reliving and releasing of an emotional experience does not necessarily cause a miraculous cure. Again quoting from Sandison's article: "It would be a mistake to suppose that all such experiences [abreactions] bring about an immediate cessation of neurotic symptoms. Obsessional neurotics in particular *can be made worse for a time*. For these patients . . . everything depends on whether they can come to terms with their repressed memories, as they emerge into consciousness. This is not always possible, but we can definitely claim that LSD-25 is of the greatest value in the classical obsessional neurosis. Provided treatment is sufficiently prolonged, our results suggest that most cases will be relieved or cured." [8] So it was, with me.

To recapitulate: Under the dual awareness of LSD, one may see extraordinary imagery and fantasy which can be interpreted symbolically; one may hear himself speak isolated and apparently meaningless words which, if pursued, may lead to forgotten and meaningful episodes; one can relive with intense emotion painful experiences which have been totally forgotten; or one can somehow, with some part of himself, become the child he has been. This last is a remarkable phenomenon, as yet not understood. It is as if one enters a region where the past and the present coexist; where time, as we know it, has no existence.

In exploring the nature of the unconscious, we found that it has been called a region of timelessness, in which vivid imagery and symbols may appear that can be interpreted; in which is contained every experience of every individual from the moment of his birth. The analogy is striking: it suggests that the taking of LSD gives one direct access to the unconscious.

LSD is not, of course, the only route to the unconscious. Psychoanalysis, as well as hypnosis and drugs like sodium pentathol, offer other routes. But those are sometimes long, circuitous, or laborious. Techniques such as dream interpretation or free association or slips of the tongue might be likened to the routes taken by a covered wagon, trekking its way across a continent to reach the ocean of the unconscious. LSD offers a non-stop jet flight.

This statement does not for one moment discredit psychoanalysis or its processes. Quite the contrary. LSD simply facilitates those processes. As many research workers have stressed, of itself LSD can not be considered a therapeutic agent. A patient under its influence may be guided into certain channels. For example, I was urged to explore and to interpret my waking dreams under LSD, just as in psychoanalysis a patient is urged to remember and interpret the dreams he has dreamed during the night. I was also encouraged to associate freely to the inexplicable words and images which bubbled out of me. I was also guided to discover and release those emotional experiences which had, without my awareness, crippled me sexually. All of these processes are standard psychotherapeutic ones used in conjunction with the drug. It cannot be emphasized too strongly that LSD is merely an adjunct to therapy, a powerful adjunct which should be administered only by skilled psychotherapists.

Under such circumstances, LSD therapy seems to produce excellent results. Several articles, written independently by research workers of several countries, have reported a high percentage of success with their patients.[9] One of these articles reports on a total of ninety-four patients given LSD, out of which sixty-five per cent either recovered completely or greatly improved.[10] Moreover, according to these doctors: "All of our early cases were either severe obsessional neurotics with a bad prognosis or were patients who had been ill for a considerable time and who had previously had prolonged treatment either by psychotherapy or other means without improvement . . . We would stress that we regarded all our cases as being very difficult psychiatric problems and that they were all in danger of becoming permanent mental invalids, lifelong neurotics, or of ending their lives by suicide." [11]

Should one herald a new miracle cure? Categorically no.

"A novelty in therapeutics is either taken up with frenzied enthusiasm . . . or else it is regarded with abysmal distrust . . . As a young man, I was caught in just such a storm of indignation aroused in the medical profession by the hypnotic suggestion treatment, which nowadays is held up in opposition to psychoanalysis by the 'sober-minded,'" Freud said in a lecture given at the University of Austria in 1917.[12]

The wheel has swung full circle. Today psychoanalysis and hypnosis are held up in opposition to LSD therapy by the "sober-minded." Since some scientists have labeled the LSD experience "a temporarily induced model psychosis," in some parts of the medical profession a storm of indignation against LSD therapy has arisen on the grounds that it may prove injurious to the health of the patient.

In doing research, I found no evidence at all that LSD, properly administered, is harmful in any way. Nor did I personally experience any ill effects from the drug, either physically or mentally. Indeed, quite the reverse. Notwithstanding these facts, and in spite of my own remarkable success with the treatment, I do not recommend LSD therapy to everyone, for three reasons:

First: LSD therapy is still experimental. Those doctors who are exploring its possibilities are pioneering—and pioneering, of its very nature, is a hazardous business.

Second: LSD is so powerful and unpredictable a drug that it should never be taken except under supervision. Certainly it should not be taken for therapeutic reasons unless with a skilled psychotherapist. Although doctors around the world are now investigating LSD as an adjunct to therapy, they are few in number. Skilled psychotherapists are rare.

Last: The techniques of LSD therapy seem to be as varied as the number of doctors working with the drug. One particular technique, devised by one group of doctors, proved successful with me. It might prove thoroughly unsuccessful with someone else.

Perhaps LSD will one day be considered an invaluable tool in psychotherapy. Perhaps, on the other hand, it will be relegated to the limbo of such miracle cures as dianetics and phrenology. The answer lies in the future. Meanwhile, I do not recommend LSD therapy to everyone.

Why then, it can justifiably be asked, have I written this book?

Because in this magnificent technological era of ours men are forging tools with which to explore the unseen microcosm which lies within the atom, and they are forging tools with which to explore the unknown macrocosm in outer space. Now, I believe, another tool has been forged, chemically, to make possible an exploration of the unseen, almost unknown realm called the unconscious. That realm has generally been considered to be an interesting, if theoretical, abstraction. As Aldous Huxley has pointed out, a few rare souls have traveled into that realm and have returned to describe it: saints like Theresa and Paul; mystics like Boehme and Blake; writers and artists like Kafka, Swedenborg, Joyce, Bosch, Goya, Picasso, Dali, Van Gogh . . .

It is well known that at first the works of these artists were ridiculed. Even after their work was accepted, they were described as weird, grotesque, "way out." So they are, to our conscious minds. But once one has traveled way out to the antipodes of the mind, creations like Kafka's cockroach, Goya's "Dream of Reason," Blake's "Tiger Tiger burning bright," Dali's melted watches, Bosch's visions of Heaven and Hell—these become reality, a reality which exists within us but beyond the reach of our conscious minds. This reality is now made accessible to us through a chemical agency, for our exploration and future understanding.

This is for me the great significance of the LSD experience, which I hope to be able in some measure to communicate.

I have purposely limited myself to the therapeutic aspects of the LSD experience, treating principally of the personal unconscious mind. LSD offers far wider fields of exploration in that domain which has been variously called the "mystic," the "integrative," and the "transcendental." But this is too amazing a province, too little comprehended as yet, to be included here, in what is essentially the examination and resolution of a neurotic problem.

When I met for a first interview with Dr. M, in charge of the LSD project, I knew only that I wanted a glimpse of the "new creation" as described by Mr. Huxley—for which glimpse I was willing to volunteer for whatever psychological tests might be necessary. Dr. M disabused me of that idea quickly, explaining that the experiment was concerned with the effectiveness of LSD in relation to specific neuroses. Since I had been psychoanalyzed and was functioning well, I was at a loss for a specific problem—until I realized that I had never overcome my frigidity.

Although sex and LSD seemed an illogical, not to say absurd, combination, I offered that problem as an area for exploration, with the assurance that I would try seriously to resolve the dilemma. Only then did Dr. M accept me as a subject.

I was next required to take certain formal tests; and after that, Dr. M outlined to me the procedure of LSD therapy which I was to follow—a procedure which startled me considerably.

To begin with: I was told that an LSD session would last for five hours. Since I had been accustomed to an analytic session which lasted for fifty minutes, I was confounded and asked what kind of therapeutic experience could be maintained over so long a period? Dr. M answered that he did not know what particular benefit would derive from any one session—but that the experience was usually interesting and informative. (This, I was to discover, was a masterly understatement.)

Dr. M further informed me that a therapist would remain with me for the full five hours, and stressed the fact that no patient was ever left alone while under the influence of the drug. This reassured me quite a little; and Dr. M continued with details of the procedure.

On arriving for the session (with an empty stomach) I would be given the drug, in pill form, and would wait quietly for half an hour, for the drug to take effect. Then I would be asked to lie down and to cover my eyes with an eyeshade. This last was another puzzlement: why an eyeshade? Dr. M replied that it was not necessary, but since it removed the visual distractions of surrounding objects, the eyeshade helped one to see more clearly the images created under the influence of the drug.

This seemed logical. The next step did not. I was told that music would be played almost constantly throughout a session.

Again I asked why, and Dr. M answered that under LSD music seems to have an immediate and powerful impact on one's emotions. This statement impressed me not at all, for I had lived most of my life in the world of the arts, and the one art which had consistently affected me least was music. I told this to Dr. M who, in his turn, was not at all impressed. He went on with the remaining instructions.

During a session I was to report faithfully whatever was happening as it was happening. Dr. M emphasized that I was never to say "nothing is happening," for something is always happening every moment of our lives, no matter how insignificant that something may seem.

This request seemed thoroughly reasonable. And the last delighted me. I was required to write a report of everything I remembered of each session, no later than twenty-four hours after the session had ended.

As it happened, I submitted voluminous reports of each session and kept carbon copies. It is because of those reports that I have been able to write a factual, and I believe accurate, description of the step-by-step therapy.

Dr. M concluded the interview by setting a day and hour for my first LSD session. I arrived promptly—if apprehensively— at the appointed time. At the end of that first session, I knew that I had traveled deep into the unconscious, a realm which I had not really believed existed. At the end of nine sessions, over a period of nine weeks, I was cured of my hitherto incurable frigidity. And at the end of five months, I felt that I had been reconstituted as a human being. I have continued to feel that way ever since.

What follows is an intimate, perhaps too intimate, account of my travels and travails under LSD therapy.

II

The Case History

4.

The Closed-Up Clam

ARRIVING promptly at Dr. M's office, I was given three small blue pills, no larger than saccharine tablets, which I swallowed down with some water out of a paper cup—a prosaic passage into the unconscious. Even more prosaic was the suggestion that I look through some magazines during the half-hour required for the drug to take effect.

For about fifteen minutes I leafed through a digest, feeling so normal I began to worry lest I was one of the small percentage of persons on whom the drug has no effect. A few moments later I became aware of the smell of gas (the kind used by dentists for oral surgery) which dissipated almost as soon as I noticed it. I wondered briefly about that vagrant odor but then decided it must have wafted in from the next suite of offices, which housed a group of dentists. I had particularly noticed those offices because I had a fear of dentists, accumulated steadily over the years. Having found a nice and natural reason for the smell, I promptly forgot about it.

At the end of the half-hour I felt a slight dizziness, as if I had had a bit too much to drink. It was then that Dr. M joined me. He asked me to lie down on the couch and gave me an eye-shade to put on. Feeling rather foolish, I put it on and lay down, whereupon Dr. M covered me with a blanket. The blanket seemed unnecessary but I accepted it without comment. I could hear Dr. M adjust the record player and after a moment symphonic music filled the room. The music seemed unnecessary too, and I told Dr. M so. I explained, cheerfully, that I was a moron musically; my tastes were limited to *un*progressive jazz like show tunes and torch songs; if Dr. M expected classical music to evoke any emotional response in me he would be disappointed. Dr. M ignored my remark and continued to play various kinds of classical music throughout this session and all of the sessions to come.

I lay for some time expecting something visually interesting, strange, to appear in my mind's eye. Nothing did. I saw only the grayish-black which I usually see when my eyes are closed. At length Dr. M asked me what was happening.

"Nothing."

"Please don't say 'nothing,' " Dr. M reminded me.

"Sorry!"

I struggled to feel or remember any sensation I might have had since taking the drug. The only thing that came to mind was the momentary smell of gas. Feeling rather foolish, I reported it. Almost immediately the smell returned. Powerfully. Dr. M asked what the smell of nitrous oxide might mean to me. I did not know, except that over the years my teeth had grown so acutely sensitive (only at the dentist's office), I could not endure even a prophylaxis without being given gas. More recently I had permitted the substitution of a powerful tranquilizer, in addition to novocaine salve rubbed over my gums and teeth. As I talked the smell of gas so intensified that I felt it would anesthetize me. Dr. M suggested that I let it anesthetize me. I tried but instead of blacking out I found myself suspended in a kind of gray-black limbo. Eventually Dr. M asked again: "What's happening?"

I did not want to say "nothing" again. I searched for some mental impression, emotional reaction, physical response. Anything. Finally, lamely: "Well . . . my left knee is twitching."

"Let it twitch."

Feeling extremely foolish, I let it twitch. After a moment my

other knee began to twitch. Then my legs started to twitch
. . . more than that . . . they began to shake . . . and so
did my arms. Before I could report what was certainly a visible
phenomenon, my whole body was shaking. Violently. *Of itself.*
Extraordinary sensation: it was as if I were observing this reaction of my body dispassionately, even curiously.

"Why am I shaking like this?" I asked Dr. M or myself or
my body, which was still shaking violently.

For answer, my teeth began to chatter. Why? Because I was
cold. Suddenly, unexpectedly, I was very very cold. Through
my chattering teeth I told Dr. M that I was freezing and
would like another blanket.

"Let yourself freeze," he replied.

The conscious part of me (which was quite disconnected
from my shaking, shivering body) began to laugh then because
what was happening was so funny and so Freudian . . . ! The
specific problem I had set for myself was of course my *frigidity:*
and here I was, quite literally *frigid.* It was too pat, too pat and
too funny——

But the cold was so real. So very real that I heard winds
roaring around me. Wild winds. Somehow I was caught up in
one of those wild whirlpools of wind. . . . I could see my
body swirling off into space . . . caught up in the very vortex
of a whirlwind . . . growing smaller and smaller . . . microscopic . . . as if all the space within the atoms of me had been
swept away in the wind. . . .

But the wind had somehow now become . . .

. . . water . . .

. . . yes . . . I was in a great whirling water . . . sinking
deeper and deeper down . . . rather a lovely sensation, being
drawn into the depths of this dark dark ocean . . . down to
the very bottom. But there I lost myself. I looked curiously
around the ocean floor to see if I could find myself. I could and
did. I was——

——a clam.

One closed-up clam, alone, at the bottom of the sea.

I heard myself laughing loudly: it was so funny and Freudian again. I was one closed-up clam, which was of course another expression of frigidity. Closed-up, non-feeling——

Dr. M cut sharply through my laughter:

"Why do you see yourself as a closed-up clam?"

My laughter aborted. The conscious part of me realized that Dr. M had asked a pertinent question for which I had no answer. Why *did* I see myself as a closed-up clam? I waited, half-expecting some new imagery to furnish forth the answer. I saw nothing but gray-black, for what seemed an endless time.

Unexpectedly Dr. M removed my eyeshade and asked me to look into the mirror he was holding in his hand. I refused, almost wildly—and shut my eyes tight. Dr. M asked again that I look into the mirror and I heard myself cry out:

"I won't look at myself! And you can't force me to open my eyes. I hate my face and I won't look at it, I won't, I won't!!"

(Only several weeks later did the full impact of this episode hit me. One of the chief purposes of psychotherapy is to look at one's self, to discover one's self. In the symbolic form of looking at my face in a mirror I had refused, even to the point of shutting my eyes tight. Literally.)

Dr. M took the mirror away and I replaced the eyeshade. Silence until Dr. M asked: "Why do you hate yourself?"

"I don't hate myself. I just . . ."

"You just what?"

"I just . . . don't know how to love. That's the big twentieth century sickness, isn't it? People can't love. Psychiatrists' cliché number one. And psychiatrists' cliché number two: if you can't love yourself, you can't love anyone else."

I realized I was jibing at Dr. M. Why? I had come for his help. Even as the conscious part of me thought this, I heard the other part of me go on in a tirade against psychotherapists and their pigeonhole terminology. *Labels for everything, cures for nothing.* When my resentment had spent itself, Dr. M commented that I had probably spent my life in intellectual rather than emotional exercise. I snapped back that I had come to him with exactly that problem which a great many people have. But not everyone. Not my husband. My husband had known how to love. He had always been there for me, full of love and understanding. He had been a rock. A rock.

Crazy unexpected laughter came welling up out of me and then I said: "Yes, he was a rock. A rock, all soft inside with cancer."

I gasped at what had surged up from the unconscious part of me. As a writer, writing with only conscious awareness, I would never have found those words.

I went on to speak of my husband's sudden swift death of a cancer no one had suspected. He had always seemed so strong. But within him, obviously, the pressures of his life had been too severe. For many of those pressures I had to accept the guilt. . . .

As I spoke, pain. Terrible pain which after a time localized in my breasts. I understood the relationship between this pain and my husband's death. I felt guilty for his death and wanted to die of cancer too. As retribution.

Dr. M asked me not to intellectualize but to "go with" the pain and see where it would lead. For a long time the pain remained static in a void of gray-blackness. Gradually an image took shape in the gray-blackness: a white marble statue of a nude woman with two gaping holes where her breasts should be; through those gaping holes shone a brilliant blue sky.

I felt as if I recognized that statue. . . . Had I seen it somewhere? . . . No . . . I remembered now . . . someone had told me that after the Second World War, there had been erected in the center of a German city, totally blitzed . . . a huge statue, visible from every part of the city . . . of a woman with gaping holes instead of breasts. The statue had been christened The City without a Heart.

I understood now. This image I had created in fantasy was meant to be a symbol of—myself. I was a Woman without a Heart, who could feel neither love nor sex.

But why?

I struggled to see some sort of answer.

Limbo.

In the limbo, the music of which I had been unaware began to envelop me. Romantic music, many violins. I found myself caught up in those violins . . . which began to itch . . . itching violins? . . . yes . . . I was surrounded by . . . or I *was* those violins itching more and more strongly until . . . somehow . . . the itching became *sexual?* . . . Yes, this was a sexual itching rather like the sensation of a clitoral orgasm. Extraordinary. I *was* those violins which were also an itching and a clitoral orgasm.

(I wish I could convey how real is this sensation of becoming something or someone other than one's self while under the drug. This experience can be wonderfully pleasant, as these violins were; or it can be hideous and terrifying, as later sessions will show. But it is always extraordinary. To retain one's own identity, yet to become another being or animal or object: the process seems related to the primitive concept of metempsychosis or to the present concept of psychosis where one believes himself to be Napoleon or Cleopatra or a glass vase which will shatter if it is touched.)

This experience seemed an extremely important one which I should report to Dr. M. I started to speak—and found that I could only stutter. I stuttered a few words about "sexual itching"—and then found I could not speak any words at all. I was, for the first time in my life, vocally paralyzed.

"Don't try to talk. Just go with those feelings."

I heard Dr. M speaking as if through layers of time. I stopped struggling for words—and immediately was flooded with strong desire for—Dr. M. Oh no no. I did not, NOT want to suffer through a transference to Dr. M. I had experienced one transference already to my analyst which had been as genuine and frustrating a feeling as unrequited love. No more transferences; no more Unrequited Love!

But even as I protested I felt more and more desire for Dr. M . . . unsolicited, unwanted yet delicious sensation . . . which continued to grow and grow until . . . so unexpectedly! . . . the pressure of a full bladder cut across and obliterated my desire. That full bladder pressure intensified. Painful now. And extremely embarrassing.

Silence.

At length Dr. M asked what was happening. I wanted very much to explain but although I was now physically capable of talking, I was mute with embarrassment. I knew the reason for that. As a child I had been a chronic bed-wetter. During my analysis I had been told that bed-wetting is an indication of a strong disturbance in childhood, usually of a sexual nature. I had tried again and again in analytic hours to discover that childhood disturbance, sexual or otherwise, without success. I had never learned the reason for my bed-wetting, nor had I overcome my sense of shame about the toilet functions. Because of that still present shame, it took an inordinate time to tell Dr. M about the bladder distress I continued to feel. When at long last I reported it, I heard a question leap out of me, totally unpremeditated:

"Is an orgasm like *wetting* someone? Is that why I don't have an orgasm?"

"I don't know. Is that why?"

Gray blankness again. I tried to find an answer to the question in the blankness but none came. Gradually the full-bladder distress dissipated and I was left, emotionless, in a gray-black void.

And then I was told that the session had ended.

I could not believe five hours had passed, yet I felt I had been living in eternity. I was to discover that this elasticity of time is one of the most distinctive features of the LSD experience. Einstein's relativity becomes the fact: a minute seems endless while five hours pass in a trice.

I left Dr. M in a state of enchantment: the intervening week seemed hardly enough to classify and comprehend the wealth of imagery and sensation which had appeared in this five-hour trice.

That evening I tried to recapitulate what had happened. Physically I had experienced violent tremors, extreme cold, clitoral "itching," intense pain in my breasts, and the acute distress of a full bladder. All of these sensations had been more real than real, yet each of them had evaporated as swiftly as they had appeared. That in itself was remarkable.

Even more remarkable was the fact that several times during the session I had heard myself say things I had not even imagined. It was as if I had been split into two entities, each with its own awareness, both operating simultaneously. The nearest analogy I could make was that of being both the audience and the actor in a surrealist film.

As I was sinking into sleep, a fleeting worry brushed past: would I remember the manifold events of the day, or would they have dissolved into the vague and unreal stuff of which dreams are made . . . ?

The next afternoon, writing the report, I found that I could remember the most trifling details of the experience. In fact, some of the imagery had become more clear and meaningful. For example: those winds of intense cold, the closed-up clam, and the statue of a City without a Heart. These were three explicit expressions of my frigidity. Each—oddly—contained a play on words. I was "cold"; I had "clammed up" against feeling; and I was "without a heart." This last image, derived from a statue which had been erected in the center of a blitzed city, was also a fine symbol for my life whose center had been blitzed when my husband died, leaving me with no capacity (or so I had thought) to earn a living for my children and myself.

Yes, these three were clear. The rest of what had happened was not. Why that smell of gas which had appeared briefly when I was alone and then returned so powerfully when Dr. M had joined me? I had been reminded of my fear of dentists and my acutely sensitive teeth—but had been stranded, just there. All during the week I puzzled over that smell of nitrous oxide, only to dismiss it as a natural association to the dentists' suite next door to Dr. M's office. Four sessions later I was to discover how wrong I was so to explain the phenomenon.

Nor did I at all understand those "itching clitoral violins" which had leaped out at me. A nice bit of surrealism. But what did it mean??

In the next days I developed an itch around my genital area. With remarkable obtuseness I did not connect this physical itching with those surrealist itching violins. The itch persisted, and a vague rash developed, both of which became so annoying that I went to the family doctor for relief. He did not recognize the rash and suggested I might have developed an allergy to the chlorine in swimming pools—although he was puzzled as to why the rash should have developed in just that one area. In any event, he prescribed a salve for the rash and some pills to stop the incessant itch, neither of which helped. About four weeks later both the rash and the itch went away—but it was not until the tenth session of therapy that I learned the reason for this quirk in my psyche which had expressed itself under LSD as "itching clitoral violins" and in daily life as a pocklike rash around the genital area which itched continually. (It is interesting to note that I looked upon the itching rash and those itching violins as two separate puzzles until that tenth session.)

Finally, and most tantalizingly, I could not understand why those wonderful sex feelings had transmuted into the acute distress of a full bladder. I remembered how as a child I had been taken from doctor to doctor for a "kidney condition," since there could be no other explanation for a normal healthy girl of six, seven, and eight wetting her bed. For the first time in many many years I remembered how intensely ashamed I had been of that "kidney condition." I also remembered those interminable hours on the analyst's couch in which I dutifully tried to recall something, *anything,* of a sexual nature which might have brought on that humiliating weak kidney. I had finally rebelled and denied that there was any relationship between bed-wetting and Freud's "infantile sexuality," which was one of those labels I had grown to scorn. For the first time, in this LSD session, I had been shown a direct connection between my sexual problem (expressed as physical desire for Dr. M) and my "kidney" problem (expressed as a distressing full bladder). A need to *wet the bed* had cut across and obliterated my sexual pleasure.

Why? Again, no trace of an answer.

Despite these mysteries, I was exhilarated rather than depressed. So much had been revealed spontaneously in this first session—surely in the second at least one of these intriguing puzzles would be solved.

Not so.

5.

The Resistance

THE night before my second session I had difficulty falling asleep. Quite a natural reaction, I reasoned as I lay awake, because of my anticipation of things to come. It was not until three o'clock that I managed to drift into sleep—only to wake again at four, at seven, and finally at nine. Groggy from the restless night I decided to doze, just that ten minute indulgence. I woke, incredibly, at a quarter to *one*. It had been years since I had slept so late. As I tore on clothes and raced to my appointment, I explained this phenomenon (borrowing a phrase from Freud) as a classic example of "unconscious resistance."

While waiting for the drug to take effect (I had been given four little blue pills this time), I remembered—or re-experienced?—a nightmare I had had some time during my troubled night, a nightmare which I had utterly "forgotten": I found myself walking into a strange room which contained nothing but a basket. In the basket was a baby. Or rather the body was that of a baby, but the head on the baby's body was the adult head of a friend of mine. I was appalled to see my friend like that. Remembering, or reliving, that nightmare now I felt all the sick horror I must have felt when I dreamed the dream—which seemed vastly important suddenly. I determined to interpret the dream with Dr. M's help when the session began. I also planned to tell him about that peculiar itch which had been plaguing me. But as I continued to wait, my mind drifted

to other things—or to nothing. By the time Dr. M joined me I
had forgotten both the dream and the rash.

For a long time the music played and I was silent. I felt
vaguely that there were things I had wanted to discuss with
Dr. M but I could not remember what they were. In fact I
felt a great reluctance to think at all. Or talk. After what seemed
an interminable silence, Dr. M asked why, in my first session,
I had associated bed-wetting with having an orgasm.

Bed-wetting . . . yes . . . that was a problem I had been
puzzling over . . . but I hadn't found any answer to it. . . .
I would like to find an answer . . . but how? Dr. M proposed
that I fantasy wetting the bed here and now. In spite of intense
embarrassment I realized that such a fantasy might evoke a
specific event out of my childhood which would be relevant to
the problem . . . yes . . . I would fantasy wetting the bed.
I tried. No emotion, no sensation, no image. Only gray-blackness.

At length the conscious part of me grew angry and impatient.
Out of my anger I remembered that I had wanted to tell Dr. M
about the nightmare and the rash. Of course. How had I
forgotten? I started to speak . . . and found that I could only
stutter. I tried harder to speak . . . and found that I could
not talk at all. That vocal paralysis began to spread to the rest
of my body. As it did, I felt that I was being swept down into
some nameless heavy atmosphere where there were no words or
images. There the two parts of me, two opposing and abstract
forces, became involved in a grim and silent struggle. As I
watched, I knew that this was a fight to the death between my
neurosis which was determined to stay alive versus my desire to
kill it off. Which side would win? Promethean struggle . . .
out of which I heard myself laughing . . . which laughter
changed into crying . . . and back into laughter . . . seesaw
of laughing/crying . . . as if the struggle deep within me was
manifesting itself in these opposite emotions. But both emotions, or both forces, were so strong that one could not defeat
the other. Gradually I became aware that Dr. M was speaking
. . . oh . . . he was asking me what was happening. . . . I

tried to explain . . . I tried to say just *anything* . . . but still no words would come. Far worse than that now. The vocal paralysis had completely spread through my body. *I could literally neither move nor talk.* Endless struggle before I could form just one word in this wordless heavy atmosphere:

". . . Paralyzed."

It had required such enormous effort to speak the word that my body had become clammy cold, corpselike. I wondered without emotion if this battle would annihilate both parts of me, leaving me dead on Dr. M's couch.

Just then—startlingly—I heard myself ask if I might sit up and smoke? I had spoken in a perfectly normal voice, and now I sat up with a perfectly normal movement. Two or three puffs of a cigarette and I was restored to the present moment, and problem. With a little embarrassed laugh I said:

"I've been trying to tell you something all afternoon. But each time I begin, I clam up."

(It was not until I collated my reports that I found this new word-play. Here I complain of "clamming up." In the first session I had seen myself as a "closed-up clam.")

"Tell me now."

"Yes. Of course. I've been trying to tell you . . ."

Again, incredibly, I clammed up. I sat staring at Dr. M, helpless to speak. Dr. M suggested I lie down again. I nodded, put out my cigarette, and began to lie down. As I did—I was gripped with a sudden and savage terror which tumbled out in a half-gasp, half-scream.

"What's happening?" Dr. M asked.

"I'm afraid! I'm afraid—you'll *hurt me!!*"

The conscious part of me was astonished at what I had said. I had never imagined that Dr. M would hurt me. Physically, or in any other way. True, during the week I had thought about him often and resented the fact that I did. I did not want to become involved in a transference. That kind of "falling in love" was too painful. . . .

Even as I heard myself give this explanation, I knew it was an intellectual rationalization having nothing at all to do with the violent terror which had welled out of me after Dr. M asked me to lie down.

"Why was I so terrified?"

For answer, only gray-blackness. Dr. M asked me to describe that gray-blackness. For perhaps the tenth time I described it as a blackness that seemed to sparkle with pinpoints of light. No more than that.

In the gray-blackness the music began to envelop me. I do not know (and probably will never know) if this was the same music that enveloped me in the first session . . . but once more violins leaped out at me, itching and clitoral . . . which immediately reminded me of the rash which had appeared during the week. Why had I developed that plaguey itch?? Dr. M suggested I go with the music to see if an image could come to explain it. I lay back and listened and felt the clitoral itching intensely—but no image came.

Very impatient and angry with myself, I sat up again—and remembered the nightmare I had wanted to interpret. This time I found that I could talk with no difficulty. Even as I described the dream I understood its meaning. Of course. It expressed in symbols what Dr. M had said in my first session: that I had permitted my intellect to predominate (the adult head) while I had kept my emotions at an infantile level (the baby's body). I felt this was a true interpretation—but irrelevant to the present problem of bed-wetting. Dr. M suggested I lie down again and try another bed-wetting fantasy.

I did not want to. At all. The last such fantasy had produced a paralyzing battle between two nameless forces which had not been resolved. I was afraid I could not survive another such struggle. But taking a deep breath, I lay down and put on the eyeshade. Almost immediately I was assailed by a force which was far from nameless: it was pure sexual desire—for Dr. M. I managed, in spite of embarrassment, to report the feeling. Dr. M asked me to go with the desire. Gradually I began to fantasy the act of love . . . only to have the feeling and the fantasy cut off abruptly by a resurgence of that full bladder . . . which grew so distressing that I asked if I might go to the ladies' room. Dr. M thought it might be better if I associated to the full bladder. Much against my will I agreed to try . . . and promptly remembered, with the vividness of revelation, that I had been plagued with a similar bladder distress before. Shortly after my marriage, I had developed the odd habit of not being able to fall asleep until I had gotten up out of bed two or three times to relieve my bladder. Most odd habit, based on no physical need, because I always performed the usual bathroom functions before retiring. All the same the habit developed during the years of my marriage into a minor compulsion—which had stopped, unnoticed, in the years of my widowhood. Why had I developed the compulsion and why had it stopped??

No answer. Only that gray-blackness which I was beginning to dislike intensely. It continued till the end of the session, leaving me in a state far removed from the euphoria of the first session.

The next day I sat down, unwillingly, to write a report. I remembered what had happened, all right, but what had happened was nothing: nothing but paralyses, vocal, physical, and mental. Pure "unconscious resistance." As I thought those words, I realized I had thought them just yesterday morning after I had slept so remarkably late. Pause for reflection: what did I mean by "unconscious resistance"—a phrase borrowed from Freud at which I habitually scoffed?

I had first heard the term, naturally, during psychoanalysis. After one or another barren stretch of analytic hours, I would complain that nothing was happening. My analyst would offer the explanation that I was "resisting." I would counter that I was not resisting at all; that I was anxious to co-operate and get well; otherwise I would not have gone into therapy, would I? He would agree that I wanted to co-operate, consciously, but that *unconsciously* I wanted to keep hidden the sources of my neurosis. His argument eventually struck me as a fine bit of sophistry—against which I was powerless. How, after all, could I overcome a resistance of which I was not even aware?

Well. Now I had become acutely aware of my resistance. It had kept me asleep until I almost missed my appointment. It had paralyzed me so that I could neither speak nor move. I had even "seen" it in fantasy as two abstract forces battling each other in some nameless region. Then those forces had evolved into a wild laughing/crying/laughing/crying seesaw out of the depths of me. Stalemate. Or rather, a triumph for the resistance—because I had discovered nothing of any consequence during the session.

Eighteen months later, I was to find in Freud's works descriptions of unconscious resistance which are startlingly parallel to my own experience. "Every step of the treatment is accompanied by resistance: every single thought, every mental act of the patient's must pay toll to the resistance and represents a compromise between the forces urging toward a cure and those gathered to oppose it." [1] And also: "As we work, we get a vivid impression of how, as each individual resistance is being mastered, a violent battle goes on in the soul of the patient . . . between two tendencies on the same ground." [2]

Sitting at my desk, I managed to overcome the resistance I was currently feeling about *reporting* my resistance—and I wrote up the session in detail. When I described the vocal paralysis I had suffered, I remembered with a shock of surprise that in my first session, too, I had begun to stutter, and then was unable to speak. At what particular point had that vocal paralysis occurred? Curious, I took out my first report. Another shock of surprise. I had become mute in the first session when I wanted to tell Dr. M about those *"itching clitoral* violins." In this second session the mutism had appeared in a far more violent form when I wanted to tell Dr. M about the itching rash around my genital area. It seemed my mutism was related to it. But what was the connection? I did not know. Having made this discovery, I went on to compare the sessions—and found another interesting parallel: in both sessions I had begun to feel desire for Dr. M, and both times my desire had transmuted into the distress of a full bladder.

Why? Again no answer.

As if to taunt me, those two symptoms—itching rash and full-bladder sensation—pursued me through the week. The rash grew worse, spreading over my stomach and thighs in what looked like scattered pocks. The itching, oddly, seemed to be most bothersome during sleep, for I would wake in the morning to find myself scratching furiously at the rash. During the days the itching would come and go but it was not intolerable. As for the full bladder, it reappeared strongly in the form of the compulsion I had developed during marriage of having to get up two and three and four times to relieve it before I could fall asleep. In addition, a third symptom arrived: I would find my arms gripped suddenly in a strong, painful tension. I had known that arm tension before, usually when I was under great pressure of work. Now it appeared at capricious moments as if to show me that the reason for this tension lay with these other two symptoms deep in my unconscious mind.

As if these physical symptoms weren't enough with which to cope—I was faced with a new emotional problem. Before therapy, I had been involved in a difficult relationship with William T, who was an amalgam of the men I had always found attractive; which is to say he was intelligent, dynamic—and unobtainable. He had made it plain that our liaison was no more than a pleasant interlude, while I was convinced that I was in love with him. Now I was no longer in love with him; I no longer felt those fluttering feelings when I thought of William. No. Those fluttering feelings still came, though—unsolicited—whenever I thought of Dr. M. Which was far too often. I rebelled against myself. I would not NOT permit this ridiculous indulgence. I would NOT, NOT fall in love again with the Unobtainable Man.

Altogether, this was a disquieting week, but—strangely—an encouraging one. I felt that the recurrence of these physical symptoms, annoying as they were, were nevertheless signposts leading to the as yet undiscovered citadel of my neurosis.

I was also to find striking corroboration for this in Freud's work. He writes: "The problematic symptom *reappears,* or appears with greater intensity, as soon as we reach the region . . . which contains the symptom's etiology, and thenceforward it accompanies the work with characteristic oscillations which are instructive to the physician. The intensity of the symptom, let us take for instance the desire to vomit, *increases* the deeper we penetrate into one of the relevant pathogenic memories. . . . If, owing to resistance, the patient delays the telling for a long time, the tension of the sensation—the desire to vomit— becomes unbearable, and if we cannot force him to speak, he actually begins to vomit. . . . The symptom, we might say, is 'on the agenda' all the time . . . The symptom that has become temporarily intensified, and has not yet been explained, persists in the patient's mind and may perhaps be more troublesome to him than it otherwise has been. There are patients who . . . are obsessed (by the symptom) in the interval between treatments." [3] I was certainly obsessed by the itching and the full bladder in "the interval between two treatments." Both symptoms "persisted" and "temporarily intensified" because they had not yet been explained. Freud adds: "This performance goes on until the working over of the pathogenic material disposes of the symptom once and for all." This was true, for me. All of my symptoms (and there were to be more) eventually disappeared "once and for all"—although my full bladder "remained on the agenda" until the fourteenth session.

So I welcomed the symptoms. I was confident that I would overcome the fierce resistance that had sprung up in the second session. I believed that after the first burst of illumination which had come to me under LSD, my unconscious mind had withdrawn in panic, not wanting to reveal itself more.

But now I felt that my desire to get well was stronger than my neurosis, and that I would overcome this "unconscious resistance" in the next session.

I was quite wrong.

6.

The Battle of the Sphincters

DETERMINED to battle the resistance and *win*, I walked into Dr. M's office and took those little blue pills. Five of them this time. Good. The increased dosage would help. In the half-hour I decided that during the session I would concentrate on the full bladder until I could evoke a fantasy of wetting the bed.

Once with Dr. M, however, I found myself all unconsciously retreating behind my several defenses: I literally forgot what it was I had decided to do; I became reluctant, then incapable of, thinking; and once again it became impossible for me to speak even if I had had something to say. At length I sank into a delicious lethargy almost mystical in essence where my personal problems seemed absurdly unimportant. I stayed and stayed and stayed in that lethargy despite Dr. M's prodding. When at length he informed me that this "beatitude" was merely a new kind of resistance, I grew angry enough with him (or with myself?) to dismiss it.

Almost immediately I was assailed by those tensions in my arms, so painful that I began to cry. Dr. M suggested I fantasy the pain to see what image it might bring. At first I could see only the gray-blackness, sparkling with pinpoints of light, but I refused to accept that nothingness and deliberately pushed past it—right into extreme full-bladderness. All right. I would fantasy wetting the bed here and now, which is what I had intended to do anyhow, before all this idiotic resistance took hold. No more resistance. I would brook none of it. Oh no, not much. . . .

In attempting the fantasy, I plunged all the way back to the fierce battle between those two abstract forces, deep in a heavy atmosphere. As the battle waged, those forces centered around my urethra and evolved into two indomitable imps who blocked the exits of my sphincters. I tried to pull those imps away so that I could release my bladder. . . . I tried, tried, tried . . . interminable and futile struggle . . . until Dr. M remarked sympathetically: "This is the battle of the sphincters."

Struggle dissolved into laughter. Dr. M's comment seemed inordinately funny. More than funny. Helpful. Because it indicated that this problem was a common one in therapy, a fact which relieved my considerable embarrassment.

Refreshed, I returned to the battle. Now, in addition to the bladder distress, the savage pain in my breasts which I had suffered in the first session. With this pain a new image: I saw that two steel spikes had been pierced through the nipples of my breasts, and a steel clamp had been locked over my vagina and/or sphincters. I recognized this as a perverse crucifixion: someone or something was crucifying my womanhood. But who, what? I strained to find out . . . but could only find that sparkling gray-black . . . which remained and remained . . . imageless and impenetrable . . . swamping me with frustration. I was hapless . . . hopeless now . . . my resistance had proved too strong, even for this powerful drug . . . nothing could help, nothing . . . my analyst had been right. I must come to terms with my frigidity since I could not overcome it.

Dr. M suggested that I might be trying too hard. He recommended that I relax, listen to the music, and see what would come of itself. I was delighted with the suggestion . . . but only for a moment . . . because as I relaxed and listened to the music . . . I was once more engulfed with desire for Dr. M

. . . which when he asked me to pursue it . . . transmuted right back to that damnable full-bladder pain.

Absolute impasse.

I could not in fantasy or reality release my bladder pressure. I could not in fantasy or reality release my sexual desire. It was blindingly evident that the two problems were interwoven. But how to unravel *either?*

Same impasse all during the week. Each night my bladder plagued me before I could fall asleep; each morning I woke to find myself scratching furiously at the rash; and at various times of day the tension in my arms would add their note to the general woe. Occasionally the tension was so strong, I felt that unless I held my arms close to my sides, I would explode.

Over and above these three—feelings of love for Dr. M, so "real" I persuaded myself this was not a transference at all. Oh no. I had fallen deeply and genuinely in love.

Certainly one of the low points in the therapy—although I had not yet struck bottom.

That I had not yet struck bottom was revealed in a brief dream during this interval—but I could not interpret the dream at the time. I had still not acquired the faculty of dream interpretation without the aid of the drug. Nonetheless I made note of the dream (reason unknown), and would like to describe it here as a demonstration of how one's unconscious can show one's psychic evolution—provided, of course, one can translate the symbols of dreams. I was lounging in the back garden with a friend when I noticed that a giant snail had *crawled completely out of its shell* and was coming toward me. I was repulsed by the snail's pulpy, grayish soft body and very frightened that it would attack me. I called to my friend, who obligingly stepped on the disgusting creature and killed it. I noticed that the giant shell was still intact, but the shell did not disturb me. I knew it was harmless.

It was many months later that I could understand this dream. The snail which appeared here after the third session belongs to the same family as the clam of the first session: at least both creatures have a hard shell which encases a soft body. In the first session, I had seen a clam *all closed up tight,* concealing its soft inner body completely. After the third session, I saw a snail *crawling completely out of its shell.* Assuming the shell to be a symbol of the outer, conscious mind and the inner body a symbol of the unconscious, then one might say over the three sessions my unconscious had learned to crawl out of its shell. However, I was still so repelled and frightened by it, that I had to have it destroyed. Had I understood the dream, I would have known there was still much resistance to battle. I did not. I simply dismissed the dream as "incomprehensible and meaningless."

As usual, the night before my fourth session I was wakeful— and bladderful. Each time I got up to go to the bathroom, I was chagrined to find that I could very easily let go. *Why* couldn't I in the course of an LSD fantasy? I did not know, but I hit on what seemed a brilliant stratagem. I would not relieve my bladder during the morning. Certainly at some point during the daylong session my normal physical demands would help the fantasy. If not the fantasy, the reality. If necessary I would *literally* wet the bed. To prevent ruining Dr. M's couch, I would take along a thick bath towel as protection. This resolve made, I drifted into sleep, about four o'clock in the morning. . . .

7.

The Screams

ARMED with the bath towel I walked into Dr. M's office, determined to battle the sphincters again—and win.

It is an interesting psychosomatic fact that from ten o'clock that morning until six o'clock that evening, I was unable either physically or psychically to relieve my bladder, in spite of intense and constant pressure for most of that time.

After prolonged struggles with those obstinate sphincters, Dr. M recommended that I give up the battle since I was being overwhelmed now with frustration which in turn was creating in me feelings of panic and despair. I certainly was filled with panic and despair—but how else could I solve the problem?

Dr. M pointed out that there are several avenues of attack on any given neurosis, and suggested a new one. He asked me to relate (or preferably to relive) whichever of my sexual experiences came to mind. I promptly remembered and described, sans emotion, my first affair which had been an occasion of numbness and disappointment. After discussing that briefly I remembered the first time I had felt pleasure and achieved a clitoral orgasm—*although I had not known what it was I was experiencing.* I had literally not known that a woman is capable of orgasm. (Or had I not remembered? Surely I must have acquired that information from sex lectures, if not from sex bull sessions.) I went on to say that several weeks after experiencing that unprecedented, wonderful sensation, I decided to experiment to see if I could evoke the same sensation by myself. I found out I could. In other words, at the age of eighteen or nineteen, I had discovered the act of masturbation.

As I told this to Dr. M, I was overcome with the improbability of what I had said. It is accepted doctrine today—not only of psychiatrists, but pediatricians and parents too—that very small children go through a period of exploration when they discover, and play with, their sexual organs. Masturbation, it is claimed, "is a universal and normal phenomenon of human growth and development." [1]

But even after psychoanalysis, even under this drug, I could remember nothing of sex or masturbation from childhood. *Nothing.*

This was more than suspect. This had to be another of the secrets held fast in my unconscious mind.

How to elicit it?

I strained to see something, anything.

I saw that gray-black limbo.

With profound shock, I heard Dr. M propose that I fantasy the act of masturbation. Immediate and violent rebellion, manifesting itself in fury, arm tensions, stuttering, embarrassment, and blankness. These were familiar patterns of resistance now . . . and even as I performed them, I realized that Dr. M's proposal was perspicacious. If there had been any significant sexual experience in my childhood which I had repressed (and it is another Freudian tenet that several sexual neuroses have their roots in some such experience), then a fantasy of this sort might reveal what that experience had been. The very violence of my protests suggested that I was, indeed, hiding something.

I stopped rebelling, overcame considerable embarrassment, and began a fantasy of masturbation. Almost as soon as I did—

I was screaming.

Scream after scream after scream after scream.

Pure brute terror.

In a void.

Terror. Sex. Terror. Masturbation. Terror. Terrible terror. I strained to see what was terrifying me.

Sparkling gray-black.

I sat up wearily. I had flunked again. For three consecutive sessions I had struggled with that sparkling black limbo of resistance and had been unable to conquer it, even with all the conscious will in my world. I would never be able to crash through it. I knew that now. I was hopeless. It would be best to stop therapy.

Dr. M asked if I really wanted to stop. I did not, really . . . there had been so many glimmerings . . . perhaps if I were to try again . . . just once more. . . .

I made an appointment for a fifth and perhaps final session.

All of my symptoms—the itching rash, the arm tensions, the full bladder—continued and worsened during the week.

In compensation, one minor insight. When I wrote a report of the session, describing those screams of terror, I was reminded of a similar terror in an earlier session. When? I looked over my earlier reports, and found it was in the second session. To overcome my vocal paralysis, I had sat up and smoked a cigarette, and then began to tell Dr. M about the itching rash—only to become mute again. He suggested I lie down. As I did, terror had welled up in me and spilled out in a "half-gasp, half-scream" after which I had said "I was afraid Dr. M would hurt me."

In this session, when Dr. M had suggested I fantasy the act of masturbation, a worse terror had poured out of me in scream after scream after scream.

Terror and lying down. Terror and being hurt. Terror and masturbation. There seemed to be a connecting link between these three. But what?

Gnawing apprehension that I would never find out. This apprehension grew into panic, a panic which manifested itself in the strongest ways the night before my fifth session. I did not sleep at all—except for one dubious hour, past six o'clock

in the morning. From midnight on, my compulsive bladder
went berserk: I must have gotten out of bed to go to the bathroom at least a dozen times during the night. About three in
the morning, I started downstairs for something to eat, tripped,
and nearly fell headlong to the bottom. Ruefully, I realized
the resistance would prefer to see me injured, or dead at the
bottom of the staircase, rather than surrender.

At six o'clock, nearly amok with anxiety, I hit on a stratagem.
Dr. M's suggestion that I fantasy the act of masturbation had
evoked wild terror in me. I did not know the reason why. Very
well. I would perform the act here and now, and perhaps find
out the reason why. . . .

No terror. Instead, an unexpected fantasy of a story by the
Marquis de Sade (read long ago and quite "forgotten") in which
a father raises his daughter to believe that his seduction of her
would be the highest honor she could know.

Puzzlement: why *that* fantasy??

Instead of finding an answer, I fell asleep. When I woke, perhaps an hour later, I had "forgotten" both the experiment and
the fantasy. What is more (to show how capricious and mali-
cious one's mind can be) *I did not remember the episode until
I wrote my report the day after the session.*

8.

The Purple Screw

JUST as though the last night's experiment had never occurred, I announced at the beginning of the session that I would like to fantasy again the act of masturbation, to see if I could evoke the same screaming terror and perhaps find its source. Dr. M agreed.

No terror. Nor any fantasy. Nothing but that infuriating sparkling black.

There followed a protracted period, filled with abortive attempts at fantasies, of which I remember nothing except increasing futility and despair, as each one dissolved into gray-black limbo. That limbo was the nothingness inside me. I had tried, both in psychoanalysis and under LSD, to look within myself. I had now to admit that I was empty inside, and desolate . . . and numb, numb as I had been after my husband's death when I could neither feel nor think nor sleep nor eat. Unendurable numbness.

I heard myself say I had always felt that numbness at climactic moments in my life: graduations, opening nights, my wedding, the births of my children. Certainly always in sex. Now, finally, under the influence of a powerful drug.

This was the ultimate numbness. This was the death of my psyche.

Suddenly a quotation from Shakespeare leaped full blown from my lips:

> There comes a tide in the affairs of men
> Which taken at their flood, leads on to fortune.
> Omitted, all the voyages of their life
> Is bound in shallows and in miseries.

. . . I had never memorized that passage. Consciously I could not have quoted it. True, I had been reading the play aloud with my son just a few nights before, but I had not made special note of those four lines.

Now I heard myself say the words . . . and I understood: The *tide* in my affairs was now. If I could not take it at its *flood*, under LSD, then *all the voyages of my life* would be *bound in the shallows and miseries* of my neurosis-tight world of unfulfilled sexuality and unfulfilled relationships such as those with William and with Arthur—and now with Dr. M: unfulfilled and unrequited loves—so wasteful—so destructive——

"I don't want that any more oh God how I don't want that any more!"

I heard myself crying. Terrible crying. I had cried like this long ago when I˙was a child . . . when when? . . . I did not know. . . . Dr. M asked me not to think but to continue to cry . . . at which point I stopped crying.

It was insuperable, this defiance, this resistance of mine. Whatever Dr. M suggested, I did the opposite. Like stopping my tears just now. Like the abortive fantasies of today. Like not releasing my bladder in fantasy or reality. Like not releasing my sexuality in fantasy or reality. Instead, invariably, that loathsome gray-black limbo of my nothingness . . . which appeared again now, and remained and remained.

Dr. M asked what was happening.

"Just that . . . goddam . . . sparkling black."

"Would you describe that sparkling black?"

"I've described it dozens of times!" Very angrily. "It's always the same. Black. Gray-black. With pinpoints of light. *I hate it!*"

"Keep watching it."

I did. I found it more and more hateful . . . disgusting . . .

worse . . . it was frightening . . . because now . . . I began
to hear a *sound* in that sparkling black . . . like a buzzing . . .
buzzing . . . oh God *that buzzing* . . .

"It's that buzzing black!"

The unconscious part of me had cried out, and now the conscious part of me recognized the buzzing. It was a sound I had
not heard since I was a little girl, trying to go to sleep at night.
After I would shut my eyes . . . instead of sleeping . . . I
would see and hear that same buzzing black with the "sparkles"
in it . . . and it would terrify me . . . because I would think
I was going crazy . . . going crazy . . . Oh dear God. . . .

I was seeing that room so clearly now where I would try to
fall asleep and heard instead that buzzing black . . . or was I
there now? . . . my brother sleeping in the twin bed next to
mine . . . and the room beyond where my grandmother slept
. . . and that other door leading down the long long hallway
to the bathroom . . . and beyond, the spare room where my
uncle and aunt stayed after their honeymoon, was it after their
honeymoon . . . ?

That buzzing black!

It was so loud in my ears now, so angry, hideous . . . go
crazy go crazy go crazy . . . out of the craziness I was in the
bathroom where my brother and I used to be bathed together
when we were very little . . . was I in the bathtub now with
my brother? . . . yes . . . that time when I noticed his penis
and asked what it was because it looked like a blister or growth
of some kind . . . and after that we weren't bathed together
any more and my sister was moved into my room and my
brother went into the spare room down the hall. . . .

Reminiscence, or re-experience, dissipated into the gray-black
limbo. Silence.

Out of the silence I heard Dr. M ask if I had ever seen my
father's penis. My analyst had once asked me that question and
I had remembered an incident which I saw now, saw so vividly:
myself as a little girl standing near my father who was nude . . .
and almost at eye level, his penis which looked very large and

reddish with . . . with a purplish-colored, sort of octagonal-shaped ring around it where it was attached to his body.

"Such a strange shape, that ring . . . like a purple screw."

When I heard myself say that, the conscious part of me laughed, and I told Dr. M how surprised I had been in later life to discover that men did not have those "purple screws" because I had thought them to be part of the male anatomy.

"How did you feel about that purple screw?"

"No way. I didn't feel any way about it. It was just there."

"Keep watching that purple screw," Dr. M recommended.

In this brief exchange I had begun to feel a strange fear which now surged into terror:

"No *no no I can't I can't!* It's too *big, too big!* It'll hurt I know *It'll hurt me because it's too big to get in!*"

In fantasy I saw that the Purple Screw was forcing its way inside me, tearing me apart and ripping me, making me bloody all bloody . . .

I heard myself screaming.

Scream after scream after scream after scream of terror.

Scream after scream like a bull screaming.

Until I exploded. All of me exploded. No, not all of me.

My face and head were still intact, attached to a baby's body.

OH GOD.

That was the dream I had had of an adult head on a baby's body—crazy—crazy——

—and meaningful.

Have I been *unconsciously* terrified of sex because as a child I had thought that a man's penis, with a purple screw, would tear me apart?

With this question, a new fantasy: a man forcing a small girl (me) to lie down . . . pinning her down with one hand . . . covering her mouth with his other hand to prevent her from screaming . . . and then raping her.

(Not until I was writing the second draft of this book did I find the parallel between this fantasy of a man forcing me *to lie down while I screamed in terror* . . . and my experience in the second session when I had "half-gasped and half-screamed" with terror when Dr. M had asked me *to lie down*. I had explained lamely that "I was afraid he would hurt me"—though I did not know why. This, obviously, was why.)

The conscious part of me was crying out now, protesting because I *knew* that had never happened to me. Never.

I sat up, bewildered. Why had that fantasy seemed so real? I knew that no one, certainly not my father, had ever raped me.

Dr. M explained that a fantasy such as this was not a real memory, but rather a "psychic reality." I did not know what he meant by "psychic reality." Dr. M clarified: Sometimes, he said, our childhood fears and anxieties are not based on real experiences but imagined ones. To illustrate: I had just "remembered" an incident in which I had seen a purple screw attached to my father's genitalia. I had not only recalled this "memory" under LSD, but also in an analytic hour several years ago. Furthermore, the image of that purple screw had made such a strong impression on me, in childhood, that in later life —as I had just told Dr. M—I believed that a purple screw was part of the male anatomy.

Yet, obviously, I had never seen that Purple Screw (unless my father were a freak, which he was not). Therefore the Purple Screw had not been a real memory, a reality, but rather a psychic reality. Similarly, this latest fantasy of being raped as a small girl had not been a reality but a psychic reality. Both of these psychic realities represented my fear of being mutilated in the act of sex.

Bizarre concept, difficult to grasp: that something imagined could have as much influence on one's behavior as something real. I could follow Dr. M's argument intellectually, but I could not assimilate it. Much confusion. . . .

I was to discover that my confusion over psychic reality was Lilliputian compared to that of Freud, when he first stumbled on the phenomenon, which "might have had fatal consequences for the whole of my work." [1]

Despite the confusion, I felt I had uncovered a truth. My

unconscious terror of a Purple Screw ripping me apart and exploding me had prevented me from sexual fulfillment—even though I had learned that there was no "Purple Screw" in reality; no danger of being ripped apart or exploded. . . .

Wonderful feeling of release.

"Was *that* the reason I've been frigid? Could it really be as simple as that?? Am I cured now, after all this time?"

I was answered violently in the negative. Not by Dr. M. But by a great resurgence of those tensions in my arms, so powerful that I began to cry with the pain, and then screamed:

"TAKE THAT BUZZING OUT OF MY ARMS!"

Yes yes . . . in some crazy way those tensions were *buzzing* . . . they *were* that buzzing black . . . but *what was* that buzzing black inside my arms? Dr. M asked me to look and see. . . . I saw that an electrical buzz saw was inside my arms . . . like those used in butchers' shops . . . what was that buzz saw doing there? . . . ? . . . I heard Dr. M ask me what I wanted to do with the buzz saw.

Leaping vividly into the fantasy—the Purple Screw. And I knew what I wanted to do: I wanted to destroy that Purple Screw so that it would not hurt me any more. Yes, I would destroy it with the buzz saw. Instead of using the buzz saw . . . I saw that I was *biting* the Purple Screw . . . *biting it off with my teeth.* . . .

"My teeth, my teeth—I have *killer* teeth! That's why my teeth are so sensitive!"

When I heard myself cry those words, I sat up, shocked by my killer teeth and shocked by my fantasied act of—castration.

It was there that the session ended.

That night I was drained, devastated—and exhilarated. I am afraid I have not been at all able to convey the emotional intensity of the afternoon, which had swung me on a pendulum from suicidal depression to gorgeous euphoria. At the farthest swing of the pendulum into depression—where I had seemed to get firmly stuck—there had appeared to me (from what un-

conscious wellspring?) a vagrant verse of Shakespeare which
started the pendulum back toward the revelation of—a Purple
Screw.

True, I had dredged up that odd memory once before, in
analysis, only to dismiss it. Today I had pushed beyond that odd
memory to find terror, such screaming terror of being ripped
apart that I had all unwittingly numbed myself into non-
feeling. Had I really become frigid, because of a non-existent
Purple Screw . . . ? I began to giggle in bed; I think I fell
asleep in the middle of a delighted giggle. Finally, finally . . .
after so much psychotherapy and failure . . . I was on my way
to psychic health . . . and all because of a nonsensical Purple
Screw. . . .

The rest of the week brought further illuminations. The next
day I began my report, by describing the night before the session, when the resistance had kept me awake past six in the
morning. In an uprush, I remembered the experiment of masturbation and the Marquis de Sade story. Fortunately I included the episode in my report; otherwise I might never have
discovered (as I did only months later) the relationship between
the de Sade story, in which a father seduces his daughter, and
the LSD fantasy of the Purple Screw, *which had belonged to
my father*, ripping me apart.

A few days later, by happenstance, my thrice-yearly prophylaxis fell due. As I walked into the dentist's office, I promptly
suffered several familiar and unpleasant sensations: dizziness,
trembling, sweaty cold, and a rapidly beating heart. In a word,
anxiety. As I waited in the anteroom, I remembered how in my
first LSD session I had noticed a smell of gas and how I had
associated that smell with my fear of dentists and my acutely
sensitive teeth. Almost immediately I remembered how in the
last session I had fantasied biting off the Purple Screw with my
teeth, and how I had cried out: "My teeth, they're killer teeth!
That's why they're so sensitive!"

Sitting in the dentist's waiting room, that seemed a preposterous explanation for my panic. But all the same . . . this

prophylaxis seemed a good way to test the hypothesis, and the validity of LSD therapy. The exposé of my "killer teeth" should have lessened their sensitivity. Yes. I would make the experiment. I would refuse the usual sedative and novocaine salve, and see if the pain and panic would survive that LSD denouement.

When I asked Dr. F to proceed with the prophylaxis without giving me any medication, he was quite naturally astonished. (He had been treating me for three years.) But he shrugged, asked me to open my mouth, and put a scraping tool inside. He was not in the least astonished then, when I jumped almost out of the chair. But even as I jumped, my mind raced to an explanation. The tooth he had touched was one of the four front teeth, one of the "killers"; my back teeth would not be so sensitive. Settling back into the chair, I asked Dr. F to clean all but my four front teeth. He looked quizzical, not to say skeptical, but when I opened my mouth wide he put the scraper all the way back to a wisdom tooth, and set to work. Contentment in me, patent bewilderment in Dr. F, as I sat unconcerned while he cleaned thoroughly all but my four front teeth. When he asked what to do about those, I said spontaneously:

"Go ahead. But I warn you—I might bite down hard."

Dr. F laughed. "You wouldn't be the first. And if you do bite down hard, you'll only be biting the instrument. I haven't put my fingers inside a patient's mouth since a two-hundred-pound six-footer bit down hard and almost took off my index finger."

I laughed—but at the same time wondered if men as well as women carry around unconscious castration wishes. . . .

Dr. F proceeded to the four "killer" teeth, and cleaned them more thoroughly than he had ever been able to clean them before, even removing long-ingrained tobacco stains. He was so struck by my dramatic recovery from fear, a common malady in his office, that he asked if I could tell him what, specifically, had cured me. I told him I was in a new kind of psychotherapy. But as for the specific reason for my cure—I could not tell him, not possibly.

As a matter of fact, I could not *believe* the reason for the cure, then or for a long time to come. Disbelief or no, from that day to this, my fear of dentists is gone. I recently had a tooth extracted, under novocaine instead of nitrous oxide. I experienced no panic and a minimum of pain.

Query: Is it possible that an *unconscious* dread of being mutilated by a Purple Screw in the act of sex creates an *unconscious* desire to castrate the offending organ with one's teeth, which *unconscious* desire manifests itself in one's conscious life as hypersensitive teeth, and a phobia of dentists?

Preposterous hypothesis. Except—in my case, it worked.

Later in the week a different illumination: one evening I was leafing through a book of photographed sculptures by Rodin, and saw as if for the first time his work *L'Emprise.* I had seen the original work twice in the Rodin Museum, and I had often looked at the photograph in this book. *But I had never understood it or felt its emotional impact until that evening.* This dynamic sculpture shows a man and woman in the act of coitus —and reveals the man's sexual organ protruding through the back of the woman. A startling picturization in marble of being torn apart in the act of sex. It was the theme of the Purple Screw fantasy, and I had a thrill of recognition.

Later I was to puzzle over that symbol. I had seen "an octagonally shaped, purplish ring" as a Purple Screw. In so describing it, I had unwittingly coined another Freudian pun. "Screw" is a slang word of undeniable sexual meaning. Yet I was convinced that as a child of four or five I had not known that sexual meaning. Why, then, had I seen a Purple Screw?

My puzzlement remained for several months—until, in doing research, I came upon these passages in Freud's *Leonardo da Vinci,* in which he discusses the "false memories" of childhood:

"The childhood memories of persons often . . . are not produced until a later period when childhood is already passed.

They are then changed and disguised . . . so that in general they cannot be strictly differentiated from fantasies. Some trace of the past was misunderstood and interpreted in the sense of the present." [2]

In the "false memory" of the Purple Screw, I believe as a child I had seen my father in the nude—but with normal genitalia. Much later, I had "misunderstood that trace of the past" and "interpreted it in the sense of the present." In other words, I must have "changed and disguised" the memory of my father's nudeness to include the Purple Screw.

Freud concludes by saying: "As a rule the memory remnants which [the patient] himself does not understand conceal invaluable evidences of the most important features of his psychic development." Certainly my "memory remnant" concealed the "invaluable evidence" that a Purple Screw attached to the male genitalia would "tear me apart and explode me." As will be blazingly clear in later sessions, the Purple Screw was a prelude to similar but far more devastating images.

Over and above these things, I developed a new pattern of behavior during the week. I found myself repeatedly tuning in to the radio station playing only classical music and enjoying it very much. This, despite the fact that I had thought I was unaffected by the music which played continuously through each session. At the end of one such afternoon I even remembered commenting, as a joke: "I've a good idea for Purgatory."

"What?"

"An LSD therapist who hates music."

But somehow in these five weeks—all unnoticed—I had grown to love good music. That love remains with me, I believe a permanent acquisition.

With this wealth of illumination, I phoned Dr. M for an hour interview, the day before my next session. I told myself I wanted to see him in order to acquaint him with these various developments . . . but I answered myself that I wanted to see

him chiefly because I was more "in love" with him than ever
. . . then I argued with myself not NOT to give in to those
ridiculous "love" feelings . . . but as events were to prove
those ridiculous feelings were far too strong for me.

In the hour, after telling Dr. M of my discoveries, I fell silent.
In the silence I became very aware of the music that was playing. It affected me as if I were under the influence of the drug.
Remarkable sensation. Dr. M suggested I lie down. When I did,
the music affected me even more strongly . . . romantic music
. . . more than romantic . . . sexual . . . strong sexual feelings in me . . . but hot on the heels of the sex . . . unexpected panic . . . expressed in those terrible tensions through
my arms . . . which I had to cross tightly over my body . . .
otherwise . . .

"Otherwise—I'm—I'm going to explode."

I heard those words come out of me, but I did not know what
they meant. More words followed:

"I'm a long scream through the tunnel."

I did not know what those words meant either.

Those two sentences were to recur spontaneously for several
weeks. They were important to the therapy. I did not know that
during this hour, however, when I explained both sentences
glibly in the light of the Purple Screw. I had seen the Purple
Screw explode me: simple enough explanation of the first sentence. Being "a long scream through the tunnel" obviously re-
ferred to my terror of being ripped apart.

Dr. M cautioned me not to give intellectualized explanations.
We would in time discover what those sentences meant. He
went on to caution me not to be too optimistic about the
therapy, in spite of the miraculous well-being I was feeling at
the moment. I had shown under LSD extremely powerful resistance, which could easily recur.

I was confident, though, that I would have no further problem with the resistance and left Dr. M, eager for the next day's
explorations.

I had now had five weeks of LSD therapy. What had I learned? Most importantly I had faced the reality of my unconscious mind, which had previously been for me an interesting but abstract concept. Secondly, I had experienced to the point of physical paralysis the reality of unconscious resistance—another concept which I had previously not accepted.

Thirdly, I had discovered the bizarre fact that an unconscious desire to bite off a Purple Screw with my teeth had been responsible for pain and panic in a dentist's office—and that the simple acquisition of the knowledge had cured me.

These three revelations had so enthralled me that I did not realize how much remained to be accomplished. Every one of my symptoms was as yet unexplained: I was still the victim of the recently developed itching rash; I was still subject to those arm tensions at odd times; and to the full-bladder distress before falling asleep. Added to these now, two strange sentences which were to haunt me: "I feel as if I were going to explode" and "I am a long scream through the tunnel."

I wish it were possible to proceed step by step, in tidy logical sequence, through the mysteries of the rash and then the arm tensions and then the full bladder and then the feeling that I was "about to explode" because I was "a long scream through the tunnel"—all the way through to my eventual and total cure. Perhaps I could do exactly that, if I were to jump back and forth from session to session, out of sequence. But that would give an erroneous impression of this therapy, which was not a continuous process. At least it was not for me. I found my unconscious mind to be an ominous buzzing black out of which leaped weird and wild things. In the next session a most savage thing leaped out at me, forcing me into new, foreign terrain.

This next session may seem irrelevant to what has gone before, and irrelevant to my specific neurosis. It proved not to be —but it was only several sessions later that these various phenomena wove together into a splendid resolution.

9.

The Cedar Chest

FOR the first time before a session I fell asleep promptly and slept soundly through the night. I woke with the sentence running through my head:

"I'm a long scream through the tunnel."

Good. It was with that sentence I would begin the session.

Both before and after Dr. M joined me for the sixth session, I tried in fantasy to be "a long scream through the tunnel." Nothing happened. I tried *not* to try: just to relax, keep the sentence in awareness, and wait for an image to form. No image formed. (This, by the way, is a discomforting experience. To try *not* to try—and to be unable to "try *not* to try.")

At length Dr. M proposed, instead of *being* a long scream through the tunnel, I *go through* the tunnel. Immediately I found myself in a long black tunnel . . . which as I explored it proved to be the inside of my brother's mouth. . . . I walked further inside . . . until I went over his uvula . . . down into a cavern of red hot fires . . .

. . . which dissolved into sparkling black.

Meaningless exploration.

Several more such explorations "through the tunnel." Each was different, each ended in limbo, each was meaningless.

Occasionally during these sorties I was plagued by a severe pain in my eyes. Dr. M asked me to fantasy the pain, but when I tried, I ended back in the sparkling black.

93

Meaningless fantasies and inexplicable pain and sparkling
black. Frustration stronger and stronger as time stretched further and further into gray-black limbo. When Dr. M proposed
that I try the fantasy still another time, rebellion and a tirade
against all these stupid fantasies which led nowhere and against
Dr. M and his stupid therapy which led nowhere—after which
I agreed to one last trek through the tunnel.

Long long long black tunnel . . . endlessly black . . . but
no . . . far far far off . . . the blackness lightened to gray.
. . . I walked toward the grayish light at the end of the tunnel
. . . and emerged . . .

. . . at the rocky reach of a bathing beach I used to go to as a
child. I hated finding myself there because I knew it was the
place where grownups went to make love and there were some
grownups making love here now and I did not want to know
who they were.

Dr. M recommended that I find out who they were.

I looked . . . and saw Dr. M with a woman, a close friend of
mine. They were making love all right.

Sharp envy, grief.

"That's what always happens to me . . . the man I love always loves someone else. Like William. Like you. Like my
father——"

I stopped. Because this last analogy was a confirmation of
what Dr. M had been maintaining: that my "being in love"
with him was pure transference. In identifying Dr. M with my
father in this fantasy, I was verifying Freud's Oedipus nonsense.

Which was patently not true. Dr. M was *not* my father.

Silence.

Dr. M proposed that I continue the fantasy. I refused. Dr. M
pointed out that my refusal was another resistance.

In the middle of this contretemps, an unexpected fantasy—
or rather, a reliving of a childhood nightmare, long forgotten:
I was a little, girl, walking into my parents' bathroom . . .
where my father was seated on the toilet, holding my brother

across his lap . . . whipping him with a strap . . . my brother was crying and his behind was all red and blue from the beating . . . and I was horrified at the sight . . . more horrified, when my father looked up at me, smiled, and said he had to do what he was doing.

Horror in me now compounded with bewilderment. Why had this long forgotten nightmare reappeared *now??* Why the *bathroom* locale which reminded me of those unpleasant bladder problems?

With what seemed considerable irrelevance Dr. M asked if I had ever been troubled with constipation. As a matter of fact, I had. Severely. But not until I was a grown woman, involved in a love affair. Gradually, my constipation became chronic, lasted throughout my marriage—only to disappear, along with the compulsive full bladder, after my husband's death.

Hearing these statements come out of me, I was struck by these two bathroom difficulties, both of which seemed connected to sex. But what was the connection?

Sparkling black.

Dr. M suggested I fantasy myself as a little girl being given an enema. I hooted derision. Dr. M's intuition was all off with *that* idea. I had never been troubled by enemas. When I had suffered with constipation I had given myself enemas often, without fear and with small discomfort. Just to prove how wrong he was, I proceeded with a complete fantasy of being given an enema as a little girl. No emotional reaction, no associations of any kind. Dr. M's suggestion was ridiculous. His whole therapy was ridiculous.

Dr. M asked if I wanted to stop therapy.

His question threw me into a maelstrom, where I cracked into a thousand pieces.

What had happened so to devastate me? I knew the answer immediately. I was shattered because Dr. M had rejected me when he suggested I stop therapy. The man I loved was rejecting me. The man I loved always rejected me. And each time I felt this shattering pain . . .

. . . *But I was damned if I would continue this behavior any more.* I would not NOT, NOT suffer the torment of rejection ever again. I would put a wall between myself and men-sex-love. And I would stop looking for a cure in this ridiculous therapy——

What the devil was I saying? I had come to the session today convinced I would find new health . . . exhilarated by all the discoveries I had made in the interval . . . yet here I was . . . proposing to abandon therapy. Why??

"Chekhov once said that if a man goes to a gambling casino, loses a million francs, and kills himself—that's not dramatic. But if a man goes to a gambling casino, *wins* a million francs, and kills himself—that's dramatic."

Like the Shakespearean quotation that had spilled out of me in a previous session, this remembered Chekhovian doctrine summed up my present predicament. I had come into experimental therapy with LSD, certainly a *gambling casino,* and I had *won a million francs* in the revelations of a Purple Screw, and the cure of a dentist phobia, and new-found enjoyment of music—but I was *going home to kill myself* by giving up therapy, and any possible chance to enjoy a healthy relationship with a man.

But what else could I do, what else? Nothing was happening and the more I *tried* to make something happen the less successful I was and the more I tried *not* to try the more sparkling black there was and there was no way out of this vicious web of resistance and already it was time for the session to end and again I had accomplished nothing, nothing, I was hapless, hopeless, helpless.

I was crying—hard, racking crying.

Dr. M suggested we continue with the session and examine why I had refused to follow up the beach fantasy, after I had identified him with my father. I stopped crying then, to fight back. Dr. M was not NOT, NOT my father in my unconscious mind or my conscious mind; he was not remotely like my father in character or in appearance; if anything, in appearance he resembled one of my sister's former beaux, a man full of erudition and no intelligence. (Only much later did I realize I was expressing hate for "the man I loved" by calling him erudite—and stupid.)

At that moment the pain in my eyes attacked again, so violently that I could not speak but only cry with the pain. Dr. M asked me to fantasy the pain. I could not.

Then he asked me to describe my sister. Difficult. At first I spoke in generalities, then focused on her spectacular courage the last two years of her life. While at medical school she contracted an incurable cancer but continued school, going into hospital for treatment during each of the school holidays. By a miracle of will, she had graduated and returned to the hospital with the word "Doctor" prefaced to her name on the door. She survived an interminable operation without an anesthetic and lived on for several weeks. I had been with her throughout the terrible summer, overwhelmed by her courage in tragedy.

When I had finished speaking of my sister, the pain in my eyes had gone.

Unexpectedly Dr. M asked if I had gone to her funeral.

I could not remember.

I could remember the hot summer at the hospital, I could remember the seven hour vigil of her operation, *but I could not remember her funeral.*

With that realization the excruciating pain in my eyes returned, blinding out thought. Dr. M cut through to ask if I could see my sister's face.

Startlingly clear image: my sister as a little girl, winsome face and smiling, mischievous eyes, so pretty. I heard Dr. M ask if I could destroy her face. Immediately in fantasy I saw myself armed with the buzz saw, attacking her face, destroying it—except——

I could not destroy her eyes.

Eyes so big—eyes—staring at me—so reproachful——

"Her eyes her eyes she asked me to give her eyes to an eye bank and I forgot I forgot I forgot——"

Savage weeping tore out of my throat as I remembered the promise I had made to my sister. Promise totally forgotten. *That* was why I could not remember her funeral. Because I had failed her.

I do not know for how long I cried. I do know that when at last I stopped, my eyes were lopsided, swollen nearly shut.

I understood then that, all *un*consciously, I had been harboring great guilt about my sister.

Dr. M added that my guilt was probably not confined to the episode of the eye bank but went all the way back to childhood episodes similarly "forgotten."

Guilts from childhood?

But I had never done anything wicked to my sister. . . . I had never been jealous of her or resentful or competitive or any of those things lumped into "sibling rivalry" . . . never. . . . My sister had been the youngest of the children . . . the least pampered, the "odd one out" . . . no . . . I did not have any guilts conscious or unconscious, I was sure of that. . . .

Sudden odd recollection: After my sister's dreadful death, I had felt so ravaged that I had gone off to Europe to recuperate. My "recuperation" had turned into a brilliantly gay holiday. Really, a celebration.

But I could not have been celebrating my sister's death? I surely had not wanted her to die—not possibly not possibly—consciously or unconsciously——

I was flailing on the couch . . . almost out of control . . . and I mumbled something. . . . I was aware of Dr. M asking what I had said . . . I did not know but I heard myself mumbling again, more clearly:

"Cedar . . . chest."

Incomprehensible. Cedar chest? What cedar chest? Dr. M asked me to keep those two words in mind.

Dim memory . . . cedar chest . . . somewhere . . . long long ago . . . my grandmother's room? . . . yes . . . there had been a cedar chest in the room my grandmother had shared with my sister when she was a baby. . . . I could see the cedar chest now at the foot of the double bed . . . but what about that cedar chest? . . . had I wanted to put my sister inside the cedar chest to get rid of her? . . . but that was ridiculous, of course I had never wanted to do anything like that. . . .

New image of the cedar chest . . . several years later . . . our family had moved into a new house where I had shared a bedroom with my sister . . . bedroom with a large walk-in closet . . . where the cedar chest had been put . . . and I had been afraid, very afraid to go into that closet *because of the cedar chest.* . . . Why had I been so afraid? . . . same fear in me now . . . and with it, the reason: I had always felt that there were *freaks* inside the cedar chest . . . freaks who would come out of the cedar chest to attack me . . . freaks, freaks . . . what freaks? . . . oh . . . around that time I had seen a horror movie about a group of freaks who had attacked and destroyed the villainess villainess villainess. . . .

Had I been afraid of the cedar chest because I had had an *un*conscious desire to attack and destroy my sister when she was little? But that was crazy. I began to protest; I knew that wasn't so, I knew it, I knew it. . . .

But it was now far past time for the session to have ended, and I was spent. Any interpretation of these long forgotten and painful memories would have to be postponed. Besides, they were *non sequiturs.* Yes. *Non sequiturs.* What, after all, could these memories have to do with my specific problems—with my being "a long scream through the tunnel" which I had originally begun to explore? Why had these crazy *non sequiturs* sprung into my awareness?

I did not have any idea. But I did have a strong fear that I might never find out; that I could not endure another such battle of resistance, frustration, and pain. . . .

Sister. Eyes. Eye Bank. Funeral. Trip to Europe. Cedar chest. Freaks. Sister. Death. Trip to Europe.

I pondered these things in the week that followed, and came to realize only too clearly what that trip to Europe had symbolized; why it had been a celebration rather than recuperation. To understand, I had to go far back into childhood (as Dr. M had suggested I do), when I had been a fat, awkward, unkempt little girl. In spite of diets, dancing lessons, acrobatics, other sports, I had been plagued with obesity and clumsiness and poor grooming all through adolescence and into womanhood. Despite these obvious handicaps I had become an actress, and a rather successful one. In character roles, chiefly. Roles in which I could disguise my own identity in the physical and emotional characteristics of someone other. All the while I studied how to make myself more attractive through grooming, make-up, coiffure. All futile.

Until that European trip which lasted a brief five weeks. In that time the ineluctable mysteries of make-up and hair-do and clothes fell into place for me. *Effortlessly.* For the first time I found myself sought after, at dinner parties and on the dance floor and as a partner.

Why?

Could it have been because, with my sister's death, I had felt *free* to be attractive?

As I grappled with this ugly question I remembered how, in contrast to me, my sister had been so slim and graceful and pretty as a child.

And then—spontaneously—another "forgotten" episode from childhood struck at me.

As a young girl, my sister had developed a serious kidney disease from which she almost did not recover. On one of the most critical of her days in the hospital I did what was for me an unprecedented thing. I went to a movie after school. In order to go to the movie, I lied to my parents, telling them I was going to the library to study. My mother went to the library to fetch me to the hospital, and of course could not find me there. I was caught in my lie and justifiably reproached for having gone out *to have a good time,* when my sister lay at the point of death.

Many many years later, when in actual fact my sister had died, I had *gone out to have a good time*—in Europe.

Here was strong evidence that I had felt jealousy and resentment of my sister, all *un*consciously, from early childhood through adulthood. I was forced to accept this truth about myself. But I could not at all understand its therapeutic value. Why was it necessary to rake up this harrowing and blessedly forgotten "sibling rivalry" which after all had nothing to do with my frigidity; with my arm tensions or rash or full bladder or that "long scream through the tunnel"?

I did not know.

And I grew more and more afraid that I would never find out. With each new LSD session I had to battle fiercer resistances before I could break through. In this last one, I had had to stay far beyond the regular hour before I could break through. Suppose no illumination were to break through at all in the next session?

Strong presagement of doom.

10.

Collapse

Doom realized.

Although Dr. M proposed various fantasies I could not or would not pursue any one of them. Hour upon hour I lay, trapped in the sparkling black.

Only toward the end of the session did a fantasy appear: I saw Dr. M as a knight on horseback, dressed in medieval panoply, surveying the field for other conquests . . . and I was the ground beneath his horse's feet. In some surrealist way, I saw that my arms and legs (which were at the same time the ground beneath the horse's hooves) were being pulled apart in four directions. . . . I was being subjected to the medieval rack torture . . . until I broke into four pieces, the center of my body crumbling, falling into space.

I needed no interpretation.

Dr. M, Knight in Shining Armor, had conquered and destroyed me and now was looking for fresh conquests. Just like the other Unrequited Loves of my life. As for me—I was crumbled, broken. There was nothing to do but to stop therapy. The drug was no longer of any help. The resistance had proved too strong. I was hopeless, abject.

Even more abject when Dr. M agreed with me. He felt that my transference was too powerful to be anything but destructive. If I wanted to continue therapy, he recommended that I work with another therapist.

Intellectually, I knew Dr. M was right: I had been fighting him more and more with contempt, ridicule, rebellion. My "love" for him was equaled by unconscious hate. And I was left, stranded in sparkling black, limbo. Yes. Intellectually I knew that.

But emotionally . . . black night of despair . . . where I discovered . . . that I could not move my right arm . . . my right arm was literally paralyzed.

Instead of being frightened, the conscious part of me was sardonic, amused. I had already experienced vocal paralysis as a form of resistance under LSD. This paralysis of my arm was another resistance. It was also a case of special pleading from my unconscious that Dr. M keep me on as his patient because without him "I had lost my right arm."

Shortly after this self-analysis I was able to move my arm again. How crafty and powerful our physiological talent to prove a psychological argument. . . .

At some time or other in this nightmare session a vague image had appeared, loathsome and evil. I had tried to describe it variously: as a reddish balloon, half-inflated and tied at one end; then as a detonating bomb with a fuse at one end; and then as a kind of purplish peapod, a poisonous peapod. Whatever the noisome thing, it faded into blackness and I could not recapture it.

I did not believe I would ever recapture it. I had finished with LSD therapy. If Dr. M who was a brilliant man could not help me, no other doctor could.

A few days later, in a deep depression, I made an appointment with the therapist Dr. M had recommended.

Three sessions later, I had worked through all those symptoms of arm tensions, rash, constipation, "the long scream through the tunnel" where I was "going to burst, or explode." And, as marvelous culmination, I overcame the specific problem of frigidity.

II.

The Purplish Poisonous Peapod

THE eighth session, and the hour interview which followed the next day, were two of the most remarkable experiences I have ever known. To convey the cumulative impact, if that is indeed possible, I am going to describe these two episodes as they happened, without any attempt at interpretation.

What follows will seem like the wanderings of a lunatic in a labyrinth leading to nowhere. Time and space are all mixed up. Now I am a woman, now a baby. I plough through a desert and I am shaken into a rag doll. Yesterday's violent pain emerges as a nightmare out of early childhood. I become a murderess, a teardrop, a purplish foetus.

And yet there is an underlying meaning behind these chaotic happenings, a meaning which I will try to convey in this chapter.

Dr. E gave me three little blue pills instead of the six I had been getting. This was depressing. If six pills had not been able to break through the resistance, how could a pittance of three? But I took the three without complaint. I was not going to complain any more. In fact, I was not going to *do* anything any more. Consciously. I was only going to see what would come of itself. If anything.

To while away the half-hour, I picked up a medical magazine which featured—oddly—several anatomical drawings by da Vinci. As I studied a splendid one, a male nude, I seemed to see, superimposed over it, that repulsive and obscene image which I had not been able to identify in the final session with Dr. M. What *was* it? . . . what had I called it? . . . a reddish balloon or a detonating bomb or . . . or a purplish peapod, poisonous . . . ?

The image persisted. Irritatingly familiar. As if I had seen it somewhere in life. But where? . . . what was it? On the tip of my mind. But before I could identify it, the image faded and I was back with the da Vinci drawing.

Several minutes later Dr. E joined me, gave me an eyeshade, and put on some music. Almost as if on cue the image reappeared, vivid and vile. Struggle to overcome my revulsion and to remember *where* I had seen that disgusting thing: *what was it?* At length Dr. E broke up the conflict by suggesting that since I hated the object so much, why did I not just destroy it?

Splendid idea. I approached the Peapod in fantasy . . . and as I did it grew larger, much larger . . . while I grew smaller, so small I was dwarfed by it. No matter. I was determined to destroy this Purplish Poisonous Peapod. I saw the dwarf that was I coming at the monstrous thing with an ax . . . hacking at it until I had chopped it into bits. Triumph. Until I looked down at those chopped-up bits . . . and saw to my mystification . . . that they had transformed into . . . deviled hard-boiled eggs . . . thousands upon thousands of deviled hard-boiled eggs . . . which now made an endless straight path leading through a desert, disappearing into infinity. To complete the scene, a brilliant blue sky shone overhead.

Crazy, surrealist, meaningless.

Derisively: "OK, doc, what am I supposed to do now?"

"Why not continue the fantasy?"

"Continue it? But it's finished."

"Maybe not. Maybe you ought to eat those eggs."

"*Eat* them!"

Barrage of protests: there were thousands and thousands of them, how could I possibly eat them all, preposterous idea, etc. etc.

Dr. E repeated his suggestion.

Thinking him lunatic but determined not to complain or resist any more, I agreed to eat those thousands and thousands of hard-boiled eggs. It would take me the full five hours and I would *still* be eating those damned hard-boiled eggs, but OK OK. No more resistance from me.

Almost at once I found that I had eaten all the eggs, traveled across the desert, and arrived at the point of infinity, which proved to be the edge of an abyss. I peered down cautiously. Far far below, grayish swirling mists . . . through which I could see ominous shapes . . . so ominous I drew back.

Dr. E recommended I go down into the abyss.

More protests: how could I possibly go down there, I would be smashed into bits, it would be pure self-destruction, suicide, etc. etc.

Just then I saw a gigantic Dr. M hovering over the abyss, forbidding me to go down into it. Dr. E asked if I were going to remain dependent on Dr. M. No, of course not.

With unexpected crazy courage (where had it come from?), I pushed past Dr. M and plunged into the abyss. Even as I plunged, I recognized the symbolism: I had pushed past the omnipotent authority and had ventured into the depths of my unconscious. This was the briefest moment of realization because . . .

. . . as I plummeted down . . . I felt myself growing smaller and smaller. . . . I was becoming a child . . . a very small child . . . a baby . . . *I was a baby. I was not remembering being a baby. I was literally a baby.* (The conscious part of me realized I was experiencing the phenomenon of "age regression," familiar in hypnosis. But in this case, although I had become a baby, I remained at the same time a grown woman lying on a couch. This was a double state of being.) The leg of the baby that I was (my own adult leg) suddenly jerked into the air and I whimpered in the voice of a little child: "They stuck me with a needle!" Before I could find out *who* had stuck me with a needle, I was playing with round, violet-colored marbles . . . which changed into squares . . . then rectangles . . . which grew long and high and became the four sides of a playpen. I was inside the playpen. My brother was outside it, playing. I whined like a baby: "They let him play outside but I have to stay in here. . . ."

And I did. But briefly. Because the sides of the playpen began to shrink . . . and became round again . . . and coalesced into one round ball . . . a violet jewel . . . an amethyst pendant . . . around someone's neck . . . whose neck? . . . I looked up from the amethyst . . . and saw my mother . . . her face purple with rage . . . shaking someone . . . viciously shaking someone . . . who was it? my brother? me? . . . whoever it was was changing . . . into a rag doll. I had become a rag doll and my mother kept shaking me and shaking me in her fury.

"STOP IT, MOTHER!"

The force of my scream stopped the fantasy. I was back to being a woman, lying on a couch, feeling utterly utterly bewildered: what had all of that meant?? Being stuck with a needle and playing with marbles which became a playpen and being beaten into a rag doll by my *mother*? My mother had never beaten me. Never. She was the opposite of that raging woman. My mother was gentle and kind. What had all of that meant?

Dr. E reminded me that I had started with an image of a "purplish poisonous peapod"——

The Peapod leaped out at me again. Huge and hideous. Gasp of recognition: It was a—penis.

But but—but I did *not* think of a penis as hideous or poisonous or loathsome or any of those things, I did *not*. I enjoyed the act of love *and* the male body very much, very much, even though I could not bring that enjoyment to fulfillment.

But if that were true—why had I seen the male organ as a Poisonous Peapod? *And* a Purple Screw which had ripped me apart and exploded me?? Those had been the two images I had seen under the drug. Did that mean that *unconsciously* the male organ was for me an instrument of torture, rather than pleasure?? I could not believe it. I genuinely admired the male body, and enjoyed it. Genuinely. Dr. E recommended I prove my protestation in a fantasy.

Straightaway I conjured up an image of Dr. M, with whom I was going to enjoy the act of love. But before I could begin the fantasy . . . I saw the Poisonous Peapod attached to Dr. M . . . fury at seeing it . . . and then I attacked it . . . hacked it into small pieces . . . and Dr. M too.

Triumph. Short-lived.

Because the Peapod reappeared, whole and hideous, on my father. Fury again, and again I destroyed it, and my father too. Again, relief and triumph.

Relief, triumph? *I had been feeling relief and triumph because I had castrated and murdered two men!*

I was a monstrous human being.

Dr. E reminded me of the original reason for this fantasy (which I had quite forgotten): to prove that *unconsciously* as well as consciously the male organ was for me an instrument of pleasure rather than pain.

Of course it was. This time I would prove it.

Preposterously in this fantasy, no matter how I tried, I could not get rid of the Peapod as my image of the male organ. After many unsuccessful attempts Dr. E gave me a hint: since I could not banish the image, why did I not fantasy the act of love *with* the Peapod?

Dreadful suggestion. Vile.

But astute, really. I knew that the male organ was not a poisonous peapod. Probably the best way to prove it to my unconscious was this very fantasy. All right. I would do it. Prolonged battle to overcome my revulsion, which I finally won. Then, as the Peapod penetrated me . . . it transformed

into . . . an electric steel drill . . . whirring no no not whirring but . . . buzzing . . . BUZZING . . . I was in that BUZZ-
ING BLACK which was going to tear me apart and explode me
just as the Purple Screw had done . . . terror of the buzzing
black . . . but slowly . . . through the terror . . . unexpected courage.

I was going to let the buzzing steel drill do what it would.
I simply waited for the pain, the explosion.

But it did not come. Instead . . . the buzzing began to
sound pleasant . . . and I began to feel pleasure . . . *real
sexual pleasure.* . . .

Sudden new fantasy: Tightly folded red rosebud. Hovering
nearby a buzzing bee, a *friendly* buzzing bee, preparing to
fertilize the flower.

Of course. That rosebud symbolized my femininity (not yet
unfolded) and the buzzing bee masculinity, which was no longer
threatening but friendly.

Wonderment at the preciseness, conciseness of this symbolic
fantasy—until Dr. E reminded me that my purpose was to find
pleasure rather than pain in the male organ and the act of love.
How had I forgotten?

Kaleidoscope of Purple Screw, detonating bomb, Poisonous
Peapod, steel drill, buzzing black . . . buzzing black, where I
had begun to feel pleasure . . . that same pleasure in me now
. . . fine . . . fine . . . I would continue the fantasy of love,
this time with an image of the male organ instead of those other
instruments of torture . . . and this time I was successful,
mirabile dictu, in keeping that image constant. Pleasure grew
in me . . . and grew . . . into strong sexual excitement . . .
only to remain there, without fulfillment.

Sensation so familiar in life. I would reach this level of
pleasure, only to be stranded there. Why, why?

"What do you think is stopping you?"

I ventured the answer that I had been fantasying an *abstract*
act of love. Now I would choose someone specific to love.
Naturally I chose Dr. M. But in this fantasy too, I was left

stranded on a high plateau of pleasure sans orgasm. What was stopping me now??

A distasteful answer appeared to me: Perhaps it was old Oedipus.

Early in psychoanalysis I had been initiated into the mysteries of the Oedipus complex, cornerstone of Freudian theory, which postulates that every boy represses into his unconscious the infantile desire to possess his mother, and every girl to possess her father. Unless the individual outgrows that phase of his "psychosexual development," he is pursued by those unconscious desires throughout his life. Many years ago my analyst had insisted I was still fighting that unconscious desire. Only a few days ago Dr. M had maintained the same thing. In the years between the two therapists, Oedipus had been hammering away all over the place. In literature, pediatrics, newspapers, theater, cocktail conversation. Even in novels of neurosis, the contemporary whodunits, "*Cherchez la femme*" had been replaced by "*Cherchez la mère ou le père.*" Oedipus is all.

I had never accepted the hypothesis. I did not accept it now. Oedipus was idiotic.

Dr. E remarked that it was *I* who had mentioned Oedipus in this context.

Well . . . yes . . .

All right. Since in this session I had determined to dare any fantasy, no matter how absurd or distasteful, I would explore Oedipus too, if for no other reason than to prove Freud wrong.

Here began another prolonged battle against the resistance which brought out all its familiar weapons: stuttering, mutism, buzzing black, limbo. I fought them all until at last a fantasy appeared:

My father burst open the door, his face distorted with lust. He strode toward me, forced me back on the couch, intending to rape me. I fought back . . . scratching at his face . . . his eyes . . . particularly his eyes . . . oh God . . . I had gouged his eyes out of his face . . . running masses of blood where his

eyes had been . . . terrible terrible . . . but . . . somehow
familiar . . . ? I had seen just that face with running masses
of blood where the eyes should be . . . where had I seen it?
. . . in a play? . . . yes, but what play? . . . a Greek play
. . . it was a character out of a Greek play but who was
it . . . ?

"Was it Jason?"

"I think it was Oedipus," Dr. E answered.

Laughter spilled out of me, kept spilling. The irony. It was
I who had insisted Oedipus was idiotic and it was I who had
created this fantasy to prove it and I had invented a scene—
for which the Greeks had always had the word.

I remembered the last scene of the play in which Oedipus,
having learned he has committed unknowingly the heinous
crimes of patricide and incest, pays retribution by gouging out
his eyes.

I had committed the identical act. Upon my father. So funny
. . . so absurd . . . so dreadful.

What did all of this mean, what was I doing??

Confusion rampant.

Dr. E recommended I repeat the fantasy. I did not want to
repeat it but I agreed. I lay back, expecting that my father
would burst into the room again. He did not. Instead—startlingly—I became the heroine of the de Sade story I had remembered a few weeks ago. I, the daughter, was being led
into a room filled with white roses, where I would know the
highest honor I could attain: my father's seduction of me——

Rebellion and rage: I would *not* accept this fantasy consciously or unconsciously, and I would *not, would not* continue it. Dr. E waited for the rebellion to burn itself out. Then
he suggested I continue this Oedipus fantasy, to see its development.

All right, all right, all right. I would carry through whatever fantasy appeared, no matter how loathsome. I lay back and
waited.

This time, as in the first fantasy, my father burst into the room and attacked me and I fought back, hacking at his face and at his eyes and at his body . . . his body . . .

. . . but . . .

Now I was in the middle of a recurrent childhood nightmare which I had utterly utterly forgotten: In a living room my aunt, a very fat lady, was seated—or rather, was propped up on a couch. Propped up, because she had *no body below her rib cage.* Her head and face, arms and breast were intact, but below her abdomen—nothing but a long piece of reddish flesh dangled in a void.

Sick horror in me: how could she live like that, without a stomach, without the rest of her body? She seemed to understand what I was thinking because she smiled reassuringly and said that the rest of her body would grow in time. As evidence she pointed to the dangling red flesh, around which now grew a new section of abdomen. She had "grown" more body, and below this new flesh, that long reddish strip dangled again. . . .

Revulsion in me as I described this nightmare I was reliving. Then, when I had done, my revulsion gave way to bewilderment: Why *this* nightmare at this particular time?? What connection could it have with me-and-father or me-and-sex or me-and-Peapod or with *anything* I had been doing during the session?

I struggled for some association, any kind of association, but none came.

It was there that the session ended.

After pulling all the scattered parts of me together, I found that I felt released, relieved—wonderful. There had been no resistance I had not been able to overcome. And, for the first time under LSD I had felt pleasure in sex, rather than terror and pain. Beyond these things, there had hurtled at me a profusion of imagery such as I had not experienced since the first session. It would take much more than the ensuing week to absorb, comprehend its meaning. Dr. E suggested I come in the next day for an hour, to attempt some absorption with him. I was delighted at the prospect.

That night, gorgeously exhausted, I fell asleep immediately and slept soundly—until five in the morning, when a pain in my eyes shocked me awake and forced me to get up to bathe my eyes. Unprecedented. My eyes had never troubled me before. Except—I remembered as I bathed them—in a session with Dr. M when I had suffered exactly this eye distress, which had proved related to the unconscious guilt I had had because I had forgotten to give my sister's eyes to an eye bank as she had requested me to do.

But why this intense eye pain *now*, after an LSD session devoted to my sexual dilemma? Frigidity and guilt about my sister. These were two distinct problems. Or weren't they——

Eventually both the pain and puzzlement subsided and I fell asleep again. On waking, I remembered the pain (now quite gone) and determined to discuss it with Dr. E during the hour.

When I met with Dr. E, he suggested I lie down, put on the eyeshade, and "go with" the music. Apparently he wanted to use the technique of LSD therapy—*without the LSD*. A bizarre challenge, certainly, and one that I was dubious of meeting. But I was willing to try. I put on the eyeshade, lay down, and listened to the music. My only response was one of inhibiting embarrassment. Probably to prime the pump, Dr. E asked if I had had any dreams during the night. I had not, but his question primed me enough to remember the pain in my eyes which, incredibly, I had forgotten in the short interval of waking up and arriving at Dr. E's office. I volunteered that the intense pain in my eyes which had wakened me was related to my sister and the forgotten promise of the eye bank.

Unexpectedly, I thought of the Cedar Chest.

Why had I thought of the Cedar Chest? What had the Cedar Chest to do with the pain in my eyes?

Dr. E asked me to tell him about the Cedar Chest. I could only recapitulate what I remembered of that LSD session (the same session when I had first felt that excruciating eye pain): that there had been a Cedar Chest in the room my grandmother shared with my baby sister when I was a very little girl; and that when we had moved into another house the Cedar Chest had been put into the closet of the bedroom I had shared with my sister; and that I had always been afraid to go into the closet because of that Cedar Chest. I did not know why I had been afraid . . . except perhaps as a very little girl I may have wanted to get rid of my baby sister by putting her into the Cedar Chest . . . but that seemed highly improbable. . . . I had never been jealous of my sister . . . ever.

All unnoticed, the pain in my eyes had come back. Now it intensified. As it did, the image of the Cedar Chest became clearer, and frightened me so that I began to cry.

"What's frightening you so much about the cedar chest?"

"I don't know—I mean—I always felt the freaks would come out of it and attack me——"

"What freaks?"

"The ones from—from that horror movie——"

In swift kaleidoscope I saw the freaks, the movie: Beautiful blond bareback rider in a circus. Her marriage to a wealthy midget in the sideshow. After the marriage she treated him cruelly. So cruelly that his confreres, the freaks, planned revenge. Climax: night, wild electrical storm. Through the rain and mud and thunder the freaks moving to attack. In awful clarity, one of the freaks: armless and legless man crawling on his belly through the mud, a knife between his teeth . . . Dissolve to a clear sunny day. The barker shouting a great new attraction. People walking inside. A *thing* in the cage on display. Like a chicken, cawing. But the face of the chicken. Mutilated almost beyond recognition. But its face, that of the beautiful blonde. Its mouth making those awful cawing sounds.

Miasma of horror, confusion, pain. Why this memory *now*??

Why this memory linked to the cedar chest, to the pain in my eyes, to my sister?

I heard Dr. E suggest I re-enact this freak movie in fantasy, using myself as the blond villainess.

"No! My mother is the blonde. She made freaks of her children—WHY DID I SAY THAT? I DON'T BELIEVE THAT!"

I shrieked protest at the spontaneous statement I had made. Only then did I realize that words and images were surging out of the depths of me without conscious awareness.

I was having an LSD reaction without LSD.

This realization swiftly gave way to an image out of yesterday's session: my mother, face purple with rage, striking out and hitting . . . who was it? . . . me? my brother? . . . I did not know but I screamed out just as I had yesterday:

"STOP IT, MOTHER!"

She stopped. I looked to see whom she had been beating. It was myself, a little girl. Little-girl Me grew smaller and smaller . . . until I was . . . a purplish *thing* . . . like a foetus or an abortion.

Miasma of horror and confusion again: what the devil had mother and Foetus Me to do with freaks-and-Cedar Chest or eyes-and-sister or with my *sexual problem* with which I had started all this insanity?

Dr. E recommended I go back to yesterday's sexual fantasy to see what any of this *did* have to do with my frigidity. OK. Here and now, while these unconscious processes were flowing so freely, I would go back to old Oedipus.

I lay back, waiting for my father to burst into the room as he had done in yesterday's fantasy. He did not. I realized I would have to look for him. . . . I did, and I found him . . . looking as he did when a young man. He did not, would not, notice me. I had to walk over to him, kiss him. Somehow . . . I got trapped inside his mouth . . . and was swept over his uvula . . . and dropped into the blackness of his stomach and intestines. How could I get out?

Choice: to emerge in a drop of semen or in a bowel movement. I chose the semen and was ejected out of his body. The semen drop I was turned into a teardrop. I was a teardrop. And that teardrop was on my face.

As I felt that teardrop on my face, I became the wretched fat little girl I used to be, who tried every conceivable way to lose weight—diets, exercise, acrobatics, sports, dancing—but who never ever grew any thinner. Fat, clumsy, unkempt me.

Sudden memory: When I was fifteen years old, I won a scholarship to study abroad. During that summer fellow students taught me how to use make-up and devised a new coiffure for me and—incredibly—I lost weight. Without effort. For the first time in my life I felt attractive, and *was* attractive to young men, particularly on the boat trip home. However: my parents met me at the dock and were shocked at my appearance. My father forbade me to use make-up and sent me to a hairdresser next day for an appropriate haircut.

That ended Attractive Me for a long time. All during college and afterwards as a young actress, I was plagued by overweight and hapless about my appearance and unattractive, so unattractive. . . .

Hearing myself say these things, I realized I had said them before under LSD . . . but when? and in what context? . . . somehow connected with my sister's death . . . or a boat trip . . . celebration . . . what *was* it?

I floundered for an answer, until Dr. E suggested it might be better to return to the sex fantasy I had begun.

Oh. I had completely forgotten about old Oedipus. Once more into the breach. . . .

Again my father refused to notice me. This time, when I approached him, he turned into Dr. M . . . with whom I proceeded to make love . . . feeling pleasure which grew stronger and stronger . . . until . . .

Dr. M and I transformed into the Rodin statue, *L'Emprise.* I was the woman through whose back the man's organ protruded. Clear dénouement. My pleasure in sex had succumbed

still once more to the pain of mutilation. I had not yet overcome
the terror of the Purple Screw.

Dr. E suggested I try the fantasy again, this time permitting
no mutilation.

Once *more* into the breach. . . .

My father remained my father. But his genitalia transformed
into a red flower with yellow seeds which somehow fertilized
me. Panic. I could not have my father's child, I could not,
monstrous idea, monstrous——

"No, it's *not!* I *can* get pregnant!"

Defiant shout from my "other voice" as in fantasy I watched
those yellow seeds growing inside me . . . growing so large I
felt that they would burst open my vagina . . . no no, not my
vagina but my bladder . . . my bladder was going to burst
. . . no no no it was my *stomach* yes my *stomach* . . . growing larger and larger until——

I saw an enormous stomach covered with a shapeless brown
skirt that fell to the ankles . . . my mother . . . my mother
. . . very pregnant. . . .

"That's my sister in there! I'VE GOT TO HACK MY SISTER OUT
OF THERE!" My other voice screamed again as in fantasy I
grabbed an ax and hacked away at my sister's foetus in my
mother's stomach.

But—blotting out that fantasy—the nightmare of my *very
fat* aunt with only the upper half of her body, her *stomach
missing.*

Now I knew. Blindingly. I must have been intensely jealous
when my sister was about to be born, and I must have wanted
to kill her off, an impulse which I had repressed from consciousness. Only to have it appear in this nightmare of a *very
fat* woman who had lost the lower half of her body. In the
nightmare the very fat woman had been my aunt and not my
mother. But I had had enough analysis to know that the substitution of one person for another in dreams (or life) is one of
the salient mechanisms of the unconscious, called "displace-

ment." I had never before seen displacement so clearly demonstrated.[1]

These diverse thoughts, which take time to write and to
read, burst in on me in one revelatory moment. All I could
do was mutter: "Holy Christ. Holy Christ. . . ."

And in fact it had been a holy experience. During this hour,
with no drug or stimulus other than music, I had uncovered
forgotten emotions and experiences of unbelievable reality.
The pain in my eyes had been excruciating—and yet it had
evaporated into a memory of a horror movie about freaks. I
had felt murderous hate and sick horror with an intensity I
had never felt in life. It is difficult to understand, if one has
not had the experience, that these emotions are not remembrances of things past. These are living, overpowering feelings
springing up from God knows where. That *where*, which only
God had known until man's recent explorations, has been
labeled the unconscious mind. For the eternity of one hour,
I had been submerged in that unconscious mind, and I had
learned that the experiences and emotions hidden there had
caused me terror of a cedar chest as a girl, a recurrent nightmare as a child, and severe physical pain in my eyes the night
before. This almost inaccessible region of mind, then, was the
true fountain head of behavior. And I might never have discovered it, were it not for LSD therapy.

Yes. This had been a holy experience.

It should be understood that I was not able to give the interpretation which follows until long after therapy was finished.
At the time of these episodes, I understood several of the individual fantasies, but I was not able to weave them into a
meaningful pattern. In spite of my lack of understanding, I
had been cured. Perplexing: how could I have been cured of
something without knowing the reasons why?

In doing research, I came upon this explanation—inevitably,
in Freud's *Interpretation of Dreams*.[2] There he writes: "I had

preserved in my notes a great many dreams of my own which, for one reason or another, I could not interpret or, at the time of dreaming them, could interpret them only imperfectly. In order to obtain material . . . I attempted to interpret some of them a year or two later. In this attempt I was invariably success-ful; indeed, I may say that the interpretation was effected more easily after all this time than when the dreams were of recent occurrence. As a possible explanation of this fact, I would sug-gest that I had overcome many of the internal resistances which had disturbed me at the time of dreaming."

If one were to substitute the word "fantasy" for "dream" throughout this paragraph (a justifiable substitution since the LSD state has been called a "waking dream"), this would render a good account of my experience. I had preserved in my notes a great many fantasies which at the time I could interpret only imperfectly. In gathering material for this book, I was far more successful at interpreting them. In fact, in the year that had elapsed the interpretation was far easier. Freud's "possible explanation" for this fact—that he had overcome the resistances which were disturbing him at the time—seems valid in my case too. Certainly at this point in therapy I had been battling such resistances that I had had to change therapists.

A purplish poisonous peapod to hard-boiled eggs in a desert to a baby shaken into a rag doll to a red rose being fertilized by a bee to Oedipus with eyes gouged out to a nightmare of a woman with half her body to terrible pain in my eyes to a cedar chest to a horror movie about freaks to a purplish foetus back to Oedipus to a teardrop to a European study tour to Rodin's *L'Emprise* back to Oedipus to my mother's pregnant stomach to hacking out my sister's foetus back to the nightmare of my aunt's half-body.

What did all these wild wanderings *mean??*

At the beginning, I saw a Poisonous Peapod so loathsome that I *destroyed it by hacking it* into bits. Those bits became eggs leading to an abyss. Plunging into the abyss, I became a baby whose mother *struck* her and *beat* her into a rag doll.

Going back to the Peapod, I saw it attached to Dr. M and then to my father. In both instances, I *hacked it up* and *destroyed it;* then *hacked up* and *destroyed* the men to whom it had been attached. Only then did I recognize the Peapod for what it was: the male organ, which my unconscious had conceived as poisonous, and an *instrument of pain.* Consciously I would not believe that, and tried to fantasy it as an instrument of pleasure. I could not. The Peapod returned, and remained obstinately a Peapod—until it changed into a steel drill and the Buzzing Black which was going to *rip me apart* and *explode me.* When I decided to permit the *mutilation*—astonishingly—I began to feel pleasure, a heightening pleasure which however did not culminate in orgasm. Trying to find out *why* it did not, I arrived at Oedipus and a fantasy in which I *gouged out* my father's eyes, and then *hacked at his body*—only to find myself in a childish nightmare of an aunt whose body *had been hacked off from the waist down.*

The night after this session, I was waked by a sharp pain in my eyes. That pain returned in the hour "talk" and evolved into Freaks coming out of the Cedar Chest to *hack up and mutilate* the villainess. The most vivid of the Freaks was the man *without arms and legs,* with a *knife* in his mouth.

When asked to fantasy myself as the villainess, I substituted my mother, who *beat* me and *mutilated* me into a purplish foetus. Here I rebelled, claiming that these fantasies had nothing to do with my sexual problem. Dr. E suggested I return to my sexual problem. I did, and became the *L'Emprise* woman who was being *ripped apart and mutilated* in the act of sex. In a second fantasy of sex, I arrived at an image of my mother's very pregnant stomach and I cried: "That's my sister in there! I've got to *hack her* out of there!" In so doing, I found myself back in the nightmare of my aunt whose body had been *hacked off from the waist down.*

There can be no doubt I had been playing on one theme over and over again in many contexts. I believe the psychiatric term for this theme is the "mutilation complex." Whatever the term, I had been expressing a strong (but totally repressed) fear of being ripped apart, mutilated, in the act of sex. At the very same time I was expressing a fear (even more deeply repressed) of my own desire to hack at, to destroy—not only the Peapod, and the men to whom it was attached—but also my sister's foetus in my mother's stomach.

Terror of destroying. Terror of being destroyed.

Before this therapy, I had not been in the least aware of either terror. Now, after eight LSD sessions, I conceded my terror of being mutilated. How could I not? Purple Screw, steel drill, electrical buzz saw, detonating bomb, *L'Emprise*, the Purplish Poisonous Peapod. Instruments of torture, all— and all sprung full blown from my own fantasies. I conceded my unconscious fear of being mutilated.

But: I still denied that *I* wanted to mutilate or destroy. Impossible. I had no such evil in me.

When at length I did admit the evil in me, it was with outrage: of what therapeutic *use* could it be to discover that I had wanted to destroy, murder, my sister—at a time when I could scarcely think? Freud has this interesting comment to make: "A child is absolutely egotistical: he feels his wants acutely, and strives remorselessly to satisfy them, especially against his competitors, other children, and first of all against his brothers and sisters. And yet we do not on that account call a child 'wicked'—we call him 'naughty'; he is not responsible for his misdeeds, either in our own judgment or in the eyes of the law. And this is as it should be, for we may expect that within the very period of life which we reckon as childhood, altruistic impulses and morality will awaken in the little egoist. . . . Many persons, then, who now love their brothers and sisters, and who feel bereaved by their deaths, harbor, in their unconscious, hostile wishes, survivals from an earlier period, wishes which are able to realize themselves in dreams. . . . I have never failed to come across this dream [let us again substitute the word *fantasy*] of the death of brothers or sisters, denoting an intense hostility e.g. I have met it in all my female patients. [Sic!] I have met with only one exception, which could easily be interpreted into a confirmation of the rule. Once, in the course of a sitting, when I was explaining this state of affairs to a female patient, since it seemed to have some bearing on the symptoms under consideration that day, she answered, to my astonishment, that she had never had such dreams. But another dream occurred to her, which presumably had nothing to do with the case—a dream which she had first dreamed at the age of four, when she was the youngest child, and had since dreamed repeatedly. *A number of children, all her brothers and sisters with her boy and girl cousins, were romping about in a meadow. Suddenly they all grew wings, flew up, and were gone!* She had no idea of the significance of this dream, but we can hardly fail to recognize it as a dream of the death of all the brothers and sisters, in its original form. I will venture to add the following analysis of it: on the death of one of this large number of children—would not our dreamer, at that time not yet four years of age, have asked some wise grownup person: 'What becomes of children when they are dead?' The answer would probably have been: 'They grow wings and become angels.' . . . Our little angel-maker [in the dream] is left alone: just think, the only one of such a crowd." [3]

I also denied that I unconsciously harbored a supreme loathing of the male organ. Even though I had seen an image of a "disgusting and obscene *thing*" which I eventually described as a "purplish poisonous peapod"—only to have the Peapod evolve into the male genitals—I still insisted that I enjoyed and admired the male body. To prove it, I tried to fantasy it as an instrument of pleasure: I was then confronted by the Peapod, a steel drill, and the dreadful buzzing black: and only then did I admit my loathing, and fear.

But this was an intellectual confession, not an emotional one. And without the emotion there is no understanding, nor is there progress.

In fact, two sessions later I was protesting—just as if these two episodes had never occurred—that I admired and enjoyed the male body. (I *did* enjoy and admire the male body in *reality*. In *psychic reality*, I loathed and feared it. There is often this dichotomy between reality and psychic reality—a fact difficult to grasp.) I said I never used the four- and five-letter slang words for the penis, because they were demeaning, derogatory. One of the four-letter words so offended me that I could never bring myself to say it: I could not say it even then, to Dr. E, under the drug. He asked what associations I had to the word. None, I answered, except that it was a synonym for the male chicken. Unexpectedly my "other voice" took over: "—And when we were children, we used the word 'cocky' for a b.m."

"Oh. Then a penis for you is the equivalent of feces."

In that same future session, I discovered the real-life context of the Purplish Poisonous Peapod which, I had first observed, was "irritatingly familiar," as if I had seen it somewhere before, in life. So I had. Surprisingly, I had seen it not as an infant or child or adolescent—but woman, of not too many years ago.

One summer evening I had had occasion to walk through a city park where, in the gloom, a man was sitting on a park bench exposing himself. In the evening shadows his genitals looked purplish and slightly swollen. This was the briefest impression because I hurried past him, rather frightened. Since he did not pursue me, I quite forgot the incident by the time I returned home. I had "forgotten" it—but the memory of a "purplish, slightly swollen" penis submerged into my unconscious mind, there to link itself to other images, like the Purple Screw and the steel drill and the detonating bomb and the electrical buzz saw.

The day after my hour with Dr. E, I found, in writing my report, additional proof (as if it were necessary) that the Peapod was actually a penis. As I typed the word "peapod," I was struck by the pun: the first syllable, pea, is slang for urine and the second syllable, pod, is something which contains seeds. Urine plus something which contains seeds: what better, more concise definition of the male organ? Puns and word plays apparently form a major pathway into the unconscious, due to a mechanism known as *condensation*.[4]

A second illumination arrived in writing the report. This one holds a particular fascination for me because I suspect in it a general principle of unconscious behavior, not yet defined. This is at best a guess. Much research would be necessary before any such hypothesis could be made.

I was sitting at my desk, facing a wall in my room, as I typed the many events of the past two days. Toward the end of the report I became aware that I had used over and over again shades of one particular *color* to describe the images I had seen—particularly the frightening images: *Purple* Screw, *Purplish* Poisonous Peapod, *violet* marbles, *amethyst* pendant, Mother's face *purplish* with rage, beating me into a *purplish* foetus . . . I looked up from my typewriter to mull over this oddity—and stared at the *violet-blue* color of the wall in my room. Violet-blue—my favorite color in decoration and dress. The color which had consistently clothed the images so terrifying to me under LSD. A coincidence? I did not know. Somehow I did not think so.

Later that day I went shopping for a nightgown and chose, unthinkingly, one of hyacinth (violet) blue. Shock of realization, after which I changed my selection to a charming yellow gown. I felt quixotic, downright absurd, as I made the switch. But . . . if by absurdity my "purple" passion was accenting or indulging my neurosis, I could try to fight it even in the innocuous affair of choosing a nightgown.

The reason I suspect there may be a general principle of unconscious motivation in one's color preference is because others in LSD therapy have had similar experiences. A friend told me that a vivid orange-and-green would appear to her kaleidoscopically before a frightening fantasy. She told me this while we were sitting in an apartment she had recently subleased. I looked up—and saw that the walls of the apartment were green, and the doors a muted orange. When I remarked on this, her face suffused with astonishment and she described her own apartment in another city which she had decorated herself: the entrance door had been painted orange, the walls green, and the furniture had been covered in predominantly green fabrics, with accents of orange for contrast.

Toward the end of the week, a third discovery. For several days I had been preoccupied with the episode I had reported in detail, of Fat Clumsy Me changing into Attractive Me when I was fifteen years old. Naggingly familiar, this transition of one Me into another. I had discussed it before in this therapy —but not in relation to the study tour I had made when I was fifteen years old. In relation to what? When? Where?

One afternoon I took out all of my reports and began to read through them, looking for the answer. In the fifth session, after describing my sister's harrowing death, I had talked of my trip to Europe to "recuperate"—or rather, to *celebrate*. Because on that trip all the problems of weight, coiffure, and grooming which had plagued me for years suddenly fell into place. I had actually written in the report: "I found myself attractive to men *for the first time in my life.*" But in the hour talk just a few days ago, I had made the same statement about the European study tour I had taken at the age of fifteen.

Twice in my life, apparently, I had made the transition of Fat Clumsy Me to Attractive Me *without realizing I had repeated my behavior.*

Why these *two* transformations, so many years apart?

After much thought it occurred to me that on both occasions I had become temporarily independent of my family. On the first trip, though, I had been too young to maintain that independence and on returning home, by submitting to the dictum of "no make-up and an appropriate haircut," had returned to childhood. On the second trip, many years later, I had been able to keep my independence. In fact, since that trip I have never been bothered by overweight or the feeling of unattractiveness.

I would like to emphasize that I achieved this cure for myself. I do believe one can achieve psychic health without recourse to therapy. It is only when one fights a consistently *losing* battle against an important problem that one needs help.

One last discovery. Actually, it was the *first* discovery of the week, arriving the night after that remarkable hour talk. I went to bed still charged with the excitement of the experience. Gradually the excitement transmuted into the sexual pleasure I had been feeling in fantasy during the last two days. That pleasure persisted, intensified—and prevented me from falling asleep.

Insight: In the weeks before, I had been unable to fall asleep because of the excitement in my bladder which had forced me up and out of bed several times each night. Now that excitement had shifted to my vagina. Perhaps my bladder disturbance was a *displacement* of sexual excitement. (After all, that odd bladder compulsion had not appeared until after I had been married—and found myself frigid.)

Was it possible that *physical sensations* could be displaced from one part of the body to another, just as emotions can be displaced from one person to another, just as identities can be displaced in dreams? I believed it *was* possible, remembering the strange perversion of foot fetishism which displaces sexual feelings from the genitals to the foot.

Well. If my bladder distress had been a displacement of sexual sensation, now returning to its proper place, that was certainly a healthy step forward. With that comforting thought, I fell asleep. . . .

12.

Venus Risen from the Sea

No TROUBLES the whole of the week—until the night before the session. I had anticipated that I would not be able to sleep. I had not anticipated that I would regress right back to the full bladder. All through the night I had constantly to get out of bed to relieve the pressure of almost nonexistent urine. At six in the morning I fell asleep—only to be awakened by powerful tensions in my arms. Those "screaming" tensions which I had almost forgotten. Why had these two particular symptoms returned? I would find out during the coming session.

While the pills were taking effect, as if on cue, the tensions in my arms returned and intensified so much that my arms began to flail about violently—*of themselves*. I had no control over them. Just then Dr. E appeared, and I cried to him in panic:

"My arms! What's happening to my arms?"

"Why don't you fantasy what's happening to them, that makes them shake?"

Chagrin. I should have known by this time to "relax, let go, and go with" the shaking.

After a moment, I saw in fantasy thousands of moths flying out of my arms. As I continued to watch, the moths changed into large birds . . . no, just one bird . . . a huge bird, like an eagle . . . yes, an eagle and now that eagle was roaring down at me, plucking something out of my body. I heard the "other voice" scream with pain, but even with the scream the conscious part of me was puzzling over the *eagle* which had *plucked* something out of me. There was something about an eagle tearing at someone's body . . . what was it?

"Isn't there a legend or a myth about an eagle plucking at somebody?" I asked.

"The legend of Prometheus. He stole fire from the Gods and was punished by being chained to a rock, and then an eagle would come every day to pluck out his——"

"Pluck out his *kidney!*" I interrupted—and then screamed again because I saw the eagle roaring down at me again, to pluck out my kidney again.

(In the legend, the eagle plucks out Prometheus's *liver*. I knew that perfectly well, but I did not realize my mistake until I wrote the report. Displacement had been at work again: I had substituted one organ in the body for another—for a specific unconscious reason which I was later to discover.)

When the eagle plunged toward me a third time I shouted unexpected defiance:

"Oh, no, you don't! I *can* steal fire from the Gods if I want to!"

In fantasy, I saw myself flying up to the sun, stealing some of its fire, and wrapping the fire around me proudly:

"There! Now I'm inviolate. *No one* can touch me!"

Even as I spoke, I realized the symbolism: I had wrapped myself in a circle of fire, and had made myself *inviolate,* so that *no one could touch me.* Apt analogy of my frigidity. (When I wrote the report later, I discovered the interesting pun in the word, "inviolate." I had made myself inviolate. And during the week, I had noticed that I was making myself *in violet* through dress and decor. My favorite color. And the color which had consistently clothed the images which frightened me under LSD.)

But *why* did I want to be inviolate, so that no one could touch me? What made me behave so stupidly? I waited for an answer. An odd one came:

I saw or remembered an episode from Joyce's *Ulysses,* in which Mr. Bloom goes out one morning to buy a kidney for his breakfast, which he cooks and eats with enjoyment, after which he goes to have his morning bowel movement, with equal enjoyment.

Why Mr. Bloom eating a kidney? Because the eagle had plucked out *my* kidney? But what—?

Kidney = full bladder. Oh. Something to do with my full-bladder compulsions? Oh god, yes. Now I was suffering that full bladder as intensely as I had last night, when it had kept me awake until six in the morning.

And now I was remembering or re-experiencing the discomfort of the chronic constipation I had had for several years after my marriage. Hell and damnation. I hated being thrust back into these toilet miseries, hated it.

Dr. E interposed that such "toilet miseries" are often a displacement of genital, sexual miseries. Of course! I had realized that very fact a few nights ago when—to my surprise—the full bladder had given way to lovely vaginal excitement. With the thought, that lovely vaginal excitement re-appeared. Wonderful relief, release. Which continued until in fantasy I saw:

Bright yellow light suffusing everything. Into it, through it, a brilliant blue sea. Dimly . . . on top of the sea appeared . . . what was it? . . . a large, very large . . . clam shell . . . open clam shell . . . and standing in it . . . a nude woman, her hair flying in the wind. As the picture became clear I recognized it:

"It's Botticelli's—Birth of Venus. Venus Risen from the Sea!"

Immediately I understood: In my first LSD session, I had been swept down to the very bottom of the ocean where I became one *closed-up clam.* Now here I was in an *open clam shell, on top of the ocean,* revealed as the Birth of Venus.

Marvelous, much too pat symbolism. Could I really have risen to the pleasures of love? I waited for an answer. . . .

But Venus remained in her clam shell, beautiful, hair flying in the wind—and she remained, motionless. I became scornful: "Oh, she's a simpering ass! She's—she's got her hand hiding her vagina!"

I tried to pull her hand away but I could not.

"I need someone to help me. . . ."

"Why not get someone, then?" Practical suggestion from Dr. E.

I was not aware of "relaxing or letting go or going with" anything. I was just, suddenly, in the middle of the music, in the middle of sex. With whom? I could not see with whom . . . but the excitement inside me grew strong . . . stronger still and stronger . . . as if my sex were expanding to become all of me. . . . I did not exist except in this exquisite sensation . . . exquisite . . . and now . . . I was experiencing what I had never before experienced . . . the ecstasy of orgasm.

So gradually the ecstasy subsided . . . until at length I was back inside my normal body . . . feeling supranormal. For the first time in my life I had achieved a genuine vaginal orgasm. Under a drug, yes. In a fantasy, yes. But that did not matter. The fact was that I had been cured of a frigidity which I had believed to be incurable.

Enchantment—until I was jolted back to the now by a request from Dr. E. He wanted me to *repeat the fantasy with a specific person.*

Staggering request. I could not possibly achieve that ecstasy so soon again! But I wanted very much to oblige Dr. E. He had given me such a magnificent gift. I would try to do as he asked: in fact, I would even go along with his Oedipal nonsense. . . .

But in the fantasy, the image of my father changed into . . . who was it? . . . no one I knew . . . a godlike being . . . whoever he was, I was with him . . . and together we were sprawled against the sky . . . and I began again to be consumed in ecstasy . . . pure ecstasy . . . but no . . . no no . . . something wrong now . . . unpleasant . . . as if . . . fear or tension? . . . oh god *yes* . . . *that terrible tension in my arms again* . . . that same screaming tension that had

wakened me in the morning . . . crawling through my arms
now . . . agony.

Panic in the agony. What had happened?

I had made a full swing from misery to ecstasy back to misery.
Why?

A procession of images, but I could scarcely see them or
describe them because my arms were shrieking so with the pain
. . . no not shrieking but buzzing . . . *buzzing* . . . that
dreadful buzzing black again . . . go crazy go crazy . . . masturbation . . . what? why masturbation? . . . buzzing buzzing
. . . buzz saw hacking off my hands and then my arms . . .
devastating pain as that inexorable buzz saw went on to hack
off my legs too . . . now I was without arms or legs . . . oh
god . . . I was that armless and legless Freak crawling on its
belly out of the Cedar Chest . . . but now that buzzing was so
loud it obliterated everything . . . except . . . what was that?
. . . black thing . . . terrifying . . . slim black thing like
. . . like a nozzle? . . . buzzing worse, pain worse . . . I was
a mass of intolerable pain . . . and out of the intolerable pain
the eagle appeared again, tearing out my kidney again. . . . I
kept screaming because the eagle kept tearing at me again and
again and I could not endure this pain any more I could not I
could not . . .

"What can you do about the pain?"

I heard Dr. E's question and suddenly I knew what I *had to
do* to be rid of it.

"I have to kill my father!"

As soon as I heard the insane cry of my other voice, I protested that I had not meant that at all, I did not want to kill
my father, hideous crime of patricide. I loved my father and I
did not want to kill him and I would not kill him ever, not even
in fantasy.

Devastating pain. Through it, I heard Dr. E suggest that perhaps I could not kill my father because I was so dependent on
him? Bell of truth. I had always been dependent on him, in
life. After my husband's death, I had become utterly numb, in-

capable of the smallest household task, until my father arrived to help me. What if my father were to die suddenly? The question plummeted up to terrorize me—and to show me that I must, I *must* conquer this dependency if I were to be of any use to my children or to myself in future.

Consciously, then, I understood the symbol of "killing off my father" to get rid of the pain. I would, in fact, be killing off my parasitic dependence on him.

With this realization I began a fantasy in which I approached my father deliberately, armed with the buzz saw . . . but . . . I could not kill him. I could not.

Long, powerful conflict in which my conscious desire to overcome the dependency fought my unconscious fear (now made conscious) of losing the dependency.

Gradually the fear crystallized—and won. I could not kill my father because he was so much stronger than I was. He would kill me first; he would destroy me just as he had destroyed me with the Purple Screw——

Monstrous image of the Purple Screw obliterating everything. In me, all the loathing and rage I had felt against the Peapod. All right, all right, all right, I would destroy the Purple Screw just as I had destroyed the Peapod. I hacked at it, in fury, until I had chopped it into bits. Then I looked down, expecting to see those deviled hard-boiled eggs. I did not. I saw instead— a tempting dish of kidneys *au madère*.

Kidney. *Kidney.*

That was what the eagle had been tearing out of me all afternoon. That was what Mr. Bloom had bought and cooked for his breakfast. Kidney. Why kidney? I did not know but I began to giggle because kidney *au madère* was one of my favorite dishes. . . .

"My favorite food. Just like violet is my favorite color. Do we choose our favorites because of these nutty unconscious emotions?"

Before Dr. E could answer, superimposed over my hysteria, a memory. When my sister had been so desperately ill as a child, it had been of a *kidney* disease. Another memory. A few years

ago, my mother had been very ill and was operated on to have
a *kidney* removed.

But what had these memories to do with *me?* I had never
had any kidney trouble, ever . . . except that "weak kidney"
I was supposed to have had when I wet the bed as a child . . .
but it had not been a weak kidney really . . . and yet . . .
these days I was being plagued by that full-bladder business
. . . but that was not a physical weakness . . .

Dr. E suggested that I look, in fantasy, to see the condition
of my kidney. I looked and saw that it was perforated, full of
pus and disease. I knew I had to get a new kidney to survive
—and I had to get it from my father.

This time I was not afraid. I attacked his body and removed
his kidney. It was a healthy one. I took it for myself. There, I
had "killed my father" and given myself a healthy new kidney.

What was I supposed to do next?

Nothing for the moment, Dr. E informed me, because the
session had come to an end.

I gathered myself together somehow. Dazed. Why all these
fantasies of *kidneys?* What did they mean, either in reality or
as symbols? I did not know. Nor did I care. Perhaps I would
find some illumination during the week. If not, there would
be next week's session. Of far more importance in this session,
for the first time in my life, I had achieved sexual release. There
was the cure. *Fait accompli.*

Most of the week I was in euphoria.

I want to make it clear that the sexual release I achieved in
the session had been a genuine *physical* orgasm, unique in my
life. That this fulfillment had occurred in a fantasy, under the
influence of a drug, was not disconcerting. In time, I reasoned,
I would achieve the same ecstasy in reality. But not for a while.
I was not married, nor was I in love (except for the unattainable
Dr. M), and the notion of sex for sex's sake—or for the sake of
a psychiatric experiment—was distasteful.

Toward the end of the week, however, in pondering my report, some of the unsolved problems of the session broke

through my euphoria. For one thing, there were those baffling kidneys which had come hurtling at me from so many directions: from that fierce Promethean eagle, from James Joyce's Mr. Bloom, from those hacked-up pieces of the Purple Screw, from my favorite dish of kidneys *au madère*, from remembrances of my sister's childhood illness and my mother's recent operation, and my persistent full-bladder compulsion each night.

I tried to find a unifying thread through this maze of phenomena but I could not. At length I took comfort in the knowledge that at the session's end I had given myself a healthy new kidney. Perhaps, I conjectured, without ever knowing what those kidneys had been meant to symbolize, I had slain that particular dragon symbol.

I conjectured all wrong. That particular dragon symbol proved to be the most difficult and painful of all my symptoms. However, since its denouement did not arrive for several sessions, it is probably best to postpone further discussion of the kidney and go on to another major puzzlement:

It was an inescapable fact that I had found glorious release —*but*—when I had tried to repeat the sexual experience, all my pleasure had transformed into crippling tensions and anxiety. *Why?*

Several strange clues: I had begun the second fantasy with Oedipus. Was it Oedipus that caused the pain and anxiety? Not likely, because the image of my father had swiftly turned into that of a godlike being with whom I had started to find ecstasy—only to have it then transmuted into those dreadful tensions in my arms, which were identical with the tensions that had waked me in the morning, and identical with the tensions that had attacked me in the half-hour the drug was taking effect. The third time the tensions attacked, they had plunged me into the buzzing black in which I had spoken odd and unrelated words: "Go crazy, go crazy" and "masturbation," after which the malevolent buzz saw had appeared to hack me into an armless and legless Freak. Finally, I had seen a blurred image of a black thing, slim and ominous, shaped like a nozzle.

Tantalizing assortment of clues to which I returned again and again. Until I found an interesting correlation in the words "go crazy, go crazy," "masturbation," and the buzz saw which hacked off my arms and legs.

Two common threats to children concerning masturbation were, in my generation: "Don't do that or you'll go crazy." And "Don't do that or (nurse, father, bogeyman, mother) will cut off your hands."

Provocative as this correlation was, it was meaningless in my particular experience. I had no memory, none, of ever having masturbated as a child. Nor, consequently, of ever having been threatened. In fact, several weeks ago, had I not told Dr. M that I had "discovered" masturbation at the age of seventeen or eighteen? I had. But in what context?

I looked back through my reports. In the fourth session, after telling Dr. M of my "discovery," he had suggested I fantasy the act of masturbation. Almost immediately I had begun to scream, and screamed like a bull, in nameless terror.

This too was provocative: the very fantasy of masturbation had evoked panic and terror in me. *Why?*

In searching for an answer, one night I decided to try, without the drug, the deep-fantasy technique of LSD therapy. I turned on the radio, "relaxed, let go, and went with" the music . . . holding the word "masturbation" in consciousness . . . hoping an image would appear. For a time, none did. Then a hazy one . . . so hazy . . . what it was? . . . slim and black . . . was it a nozzle? . . . yes . . . it was a slim and black . . . *enema* nozzle. Nothing more than that.

Enema nozzle? Just one more mystification to add to the full-bladder compulsion, the arm tensions, the recurrent feeling that I would burst or explode unless I held my arms close to my sides, the "long scream through the tunnel" and the itching rash—which had by this time faded into nothingness.

No two of these phenomena seemed connected in any way. But in the next two sessions, all of those seemingly ill-assorted symptoms (with the exception of the kidney, as I have already remarked) were to come together in a wildly unexpected—and to me thrilling—explanation and resolution.

I3.

The Slim Black Nozzle

IN SPITE of the wakeful and bladderful night I spent before the tenth session, usually a harbinger of unconscious events to come, the drug had no effect in the half-hour, and none for a considerable time after Dr. E joined me. I saw no images or fantasies. I felt no second awareness. With discouraging rationality and lack of insight, I discussed one and another of the unsolved problems: the kidney, the arm tensions, and so on. Eventually, I rambled on to the almost sleepless night I had had. Then I remembered the briefest dream—or fantasy?—which had appeared briefly and which I had forgotten. It consisted of one rather frightening image: my brother coming toward me with his hands outstretched as if to choke me.

I could make nothing of the image through associations. Dr. E then suggested I improvise a fantasy around this theme of being choked by my brother. I proceeded to have several "choke" improvisations, none of which seemed productive. (Actually, this choke-image was to return, become a symptom, intensify, and lead to an important discovery—but not until three sessions later.)

But in the last of these fantasies, as my brother came toward me, I decided I would not let him choke me again. A struggle ensued; at the end of which I saw that I had castrated him. At this stage of therapy I had castrated several men in several fantasies and I was neither horrified nor outraged until . . .

I saw that, in the fantasy, I had acquired my brother's genitals. *They were now a part of me.* Wild protests: I did not want to be a man, I had never wanted to be a man, I had *no* homosexual drives, etc., etc. None of these protests dissolved the image. In my mind's eye, I remained and remained a *man.*

At length Dr. E suggested I explore the reason why I had become a man. Wilder protests—which I recognized as resistance. But against what?

An odd image appeared: that of a nude woman whom I did not know, but whose genitals I wanted to touch. As I approached her in fantasy, she grew smaller . . . smaller and younger . . . until her genitals were no longer those of a woman but of a young girl, without pubic hair . . . the girl became younger still, a child . . . and now a baby . . . a nude baby . . . and as I approached and touched the baby . . . the baby became . . . *myself.*

Once again, literally, I had become a baby. And I spoke now in a whimpering baby voice:

"She—she—she won't let me—play with myself!"

Conscious Me was bewildered: why had I said those words? Where was I? Who was "she"?

It seemed as if I were in a crib . . . and I wanted to play with myself . . . but someone was pulling my hand away . . . who was it? I looked up and saw a woman's round face with steel-gray hair and a white nurse's cap. I had no idea who she was, but my baby voice said: "That's Miss Leahy! And she won't let me play with myself!"

"Why won't she?" Dr. E asked.

I did not know . . . and anyhow Miss Leahy was doing something else to me now . . . what was she doing? . . . was *she* playing with me? . . . no, no . . . she was putting something inside me down there . . . what was it? . . . her finger? . . . no no . . . what was it?

I was suddenly afraid, so very afraid. In panic, I clutched at my head . . . and touched all that hair . . . so confusing to feel so much hair . . .

"That's all wrong! I don't have hair! I didn't have any hair until long after I was born!"

I began to whimper and cry. From far away, I could hear Dr. E ask questions with long words in them but I could not answer his questions because I did not understand those long words but he kept on asking and asking those questions with the long words in them——

"I don' know any big words!"

"Use little words then."

"Oh . . ."

Conscious Me thought that was a sensible idea, but Baby Me still had to work hard to find even little words:

"Well—you see—I'm—I'm in my crib—and and—and Miss Leahy—no NO!"

Crazily self-propelled, my arms had flung themselves criss-cross over my chest and now I could not move them. It was as if they had been pinned into some sort of strait jacket. I fought to move my arms but I could not. I began to cry, frantically, because Miss Leahy had pinned my arms down so that I could not move them, so that I could not play with myself.

Now my arms started to ache. Unbearably ache. Oh god. My arms were screaming now with those terrible tensions. I began to scream too. Then I began to struggle. Fierce fierce struggle to break out of the strait jacket. One enormous effort—and I wrenched my arms loose.

I lay back exhausted, drenched with sweat—but liberated. My arms were free to move, and free of that terrible tension. Exquisite release and relief.

After which, rampant confusion. What had all that been about? Someone whom I did not know, presumably a nurse named Miss Leahy, had pinned my arms down when I was a baby so that I could not play with myself.

But that made no sense at all. None. I had never had a nurse when I was a baby. There had been no Miss Leahy. She just did not exist.

Dr. E asked if I could see her face again. I could, with even more clarity than I had seen it before. Round face, steel-gray hair, and on her hair a white nurse's cap trimmed with a small band of black. Dr. E told me to keep watching her face. Gradually I saw something superimpose itself over her face . . . but what was it? . . . black something . . . so blurred . . . black something, slim and black . . . I knew I had seen it before . . . but where? . . . oh . . . yes yes . . . it was that slim black . . . *enema* nozzle. But what did *that* mean?

Confusion. Until Dr. E suggested I fantasy Miss Leahy giving me an enema as a baby. Then wild protests. Which stopped because, with a ring of the truth bell, I remembered how I had seen this same enema nozzle, for the first time, just a few nights ago.

I told Dr. E in detail about my experiment in deep fantasy without the drug, and about the events leading up to the experiment. I described how, in meditating the last session, I had linked together the words "go crazy," "masturbation," and the buzz saw hacking off my arms and legs; how, in thinking about masturbation, I had remembered an earlier session with Dr. M in which I had claimed to discover the act of masturbation at the age of eighteen or so; and how when Dr. M had suggested I fantasy the act, I had screamed and screamed in nameless terror. Then, in a "do it yourself" therapy at home, I had listened to music, relaxed, and waited to see what image would come when I thought of the word "masturbation." There had appeared the slim black nozzle, which I had identified as an *enema* nozzle.

I spent considerable time explaining this to Dr. E, probably (I realize now) to avoid getting on with the fantasy. Dr. E listened politely, then repeated his suggestion.

Strong effort of will to create an image of Miss Leahy holding that black enema nozzle; stronger effort to fantasy her coming toward me with it . . . and then . . . the image was obliterated in the buzzing black. But I would have none of that resistance. I clambered out of the buzzing black and created again an image of Miss Leahy with the enema nozzle. Another protracted struggle before I could fantasy her coming toward me, inserting the nozzle. As she did . . . the nozzle changed

. . . kaleidoscopically . . . into a red-hot poker . . . into an acetylene blowtorch . . . into a buzz saw.

Terrible pain which for a moment, crazily, became pleasurable, then reverted into pain. Now Miss Leahy became a devil with a devil's mask through which I could see fiery eyes, fiery eyes belonging to my father. But then my father changed back into Miss Leahy who was again filling me full of hot hot water, through the black enema nozzle, which changed into an acetylene blowtorch.

Now a second blowtorch was thrust into my urethra. A third into my vagina. I was being attacked at all three apertures by blowtorches. I was on fire inside and the fire was consuming me. Limbo of flaming pain. Then the flames transmuted again into boiling water which Miss Leahy poured into me, and kept pouring into me relentlessly. Nazi water torture. Water pouring and pouring into me. . . . I began to swell larger and larger . . . larger still. . . . I was now a gigantic balloon of a woman . . . rising higher and higher in the sky . . . higher and higher, swelling larger and larger . . . until . . .

I burst.

Wretched anticlimax, when Dr. E told me the session was over; ameliorated when he recommended I have another session after an interval of three days instead of the usual week, so that I might more quickly work through this particular problem which he named "masochism."

Perhaps it was masochism. I did not know, nor did I care about the terminology. I only knew I hated whatever it was and wanted to be rid of it.

And I was badly shaken. It seemed my "cure" had not been accomplished after all. . . .

At home that night, I puzzled mightily over the appearance of that unknown nurse named Miss Leahy who had pinned my arms down in a strait jacket, and who had terrorized me with the enema nozzle. Since I could make nothing of the episode, I decided to talk with my mother, in the hope she could throw some light on those early years.

I was careful in our talk not to ask any direct questions, but when the opportunity presented itself, I asked if she had ever hired a nurse for her children. She answered, as I expected, that she had never had a nurse, not even when we were newborn.

I asked then if a nurse had ever stayed in our home when we were little.

"No. Except that summer when your aunt was dying."

My mother sighed deeply, as she thought of that terrible summer. One of my aunts who had suffered for years with an incurable cancer spent the last months of her life in our home. It had been an unbelievably hot summer; my mother had been in the last stages of a difficult pregnancy with my sister; and to add to the general woe my brother and I had come down with *both* measles and chicken pox. . . .

During that summer, my mother added unexpectedly, the nurse had sometimes helped to care for us children.

I felt a sudden chill.

"What was the nurse's name, mother? Do you remember?"

"Of course I do. She was a wonderful woman. Her name was Miss Leahy."

When I could speak, I asked my mother to describe Miss Leahy. According to her description, Miss Leahy had been a heavy woman, with a round face, gray-black hair, on top of which she had worn a white nurse's cap trimmed at the top with black ribbon.

I had "forgotten" all about Miss Leahy consciously. But I had remembered her, unconsciously, with remarkable accuracy— even though she had stayed with us just one summer when I was, by calculation, exactly two and one half years old.

Later it was to disturb me that I might never have learned about the real Miss Leahy, were it not for mother's testimony. It seemed like cheating, somehow, to have recourse to outside help. Other patients in therapy might not be so fortunate . . .

Again I found comfort in Freud. Apparently when he was conducting his own analysis (there was no analyst then to do it for him), he resorted to a similar device. In a letter to Wilhelm Fliess, dated October 3, 1897, he wrote:

"Outwardly very little is happening to me, but inside me something very interesting is happening. For the last four days my self-analysis . . . has been making progress in dreams and yielding the most valuable conclusions and evidence. . . . To describe it in writing is far more difficult than anything else, and besides it is far too extensive. I can only say that . . . my 'primary originator' [of neurosis] was an ugly, elderly but clever woman who told me a great deal about God and hell, and gave me a high opinion of my own capacities . . ."

In a later letter, of October 15, he continues:

"My self-analysis is the most important thing I have in hand, and promises to be of the greatest value to me, when it is finished . . . My practice, ominously enough, still allows me plenty of free time. All this is the more valuable from my point of view because I have succeeded in finding a number of real points of reference. *I asked my mother whether she remembered my nurse.* 'Of course,' she said, 'an elderly woman, very shrewd indeed. She was always taking you to church. When you came home you used to preach and tell us all about how God conducted his affairs.' " [1] He goes on, in the same letter, to give confirmations of other childhood experiences he had "forgotten" and then recovered by way of dreams.

Perhaps to provide substantiation to his claim that dreams reveal authentic events from one's infancy on, Freud quotes from an earlier authority:

"Maury relates that as a child he often went from his native city, Meaux, to the neighboring Trilport, where his father was superintending the construction of a bridge. One night a dream transported him to Trilport and he was once more playing in the streets there. A man approached him, wearing a sort of uniform. Maury asked his name, and he introduced himself, saying that his name was C., and that he was a bridge guard. On waking, Maury, who still doubted the actuality of the reminiscence, asked his old servant, who had been with him in his childhood, whether she remembered a man of this name. 'Of course,' was the reply: 'he used to be watchman on the bridge which your father was building then.' " [2]

Lastly, Kris in his Introduction to *Origins of Psychoanalysis* adds: "To obtain confirmation of a point he [Freud] asked his mother for information, and her confirmation not only helped him towards understanding his own problems, but also gave him increased confidence in the reliability of his methods."

When I went to bed that night, I was far too excited to sleep. I had, after all, made the startling discovery that the appearance in an LSD fantasy of an unknown nurse named Miss Leahy had a definite basis in reality. As I lay awake, assimilating this knowledge, it occurred to me that the other episodes from the LSD fantasies might have an equal basis in reality. With this thought illuminations burst in on me from all over the place.

It seemed that when I was two and a half years old, I had contracted both measles and chicken pox, one right after the other.

Insight: Both diseases manifest themselves as itching rashes. I had contracted an itching rash after my first LSD session, which the doctor had not been able to identify but had described as little pocks. . . .

Why had I contracted the itching rash after that first session? I remembered, suddenly, those surrealist itching *clitoral* violins, somehow sexual. . . .

Again: chicken pox and measles both itch, incessantly. I must have scratched at the itching places of my body. Perhaps one of those places had been around the genital area, and in scratching at the itch—I might accidentally have discovered the *clitoral* pleasures of masturbation—*only to have my arms pinned down by Miss Leahy.*

"She won't let me play with myself!" is what I had cried in the session. Far more probably, Miss Leahy had pinned my arms down to prevent me from scratching, and perhaps scarring myself. But as a baby, I could not have understood that. Probably I had understood my arms being pinned down as a punishment for "playing with myself"!

So dreadful had been that punishment (I remembered the fierce, fierce struggle of the afternoon, to break out of the "strait jacket") that I had repressed the whole episode, including the very *memory* of masturbation. I had believed, in all honesty, that I had discovered masturbation at the age of eighteen or so. A much greater likelihood was that I had discovered it at the age most children do (from two to three years, according to the authorities), and then had banished the discovery into the unconscious because it had been so painfully associated with being pinned into a strait jacket so that I could not move my arms.

Now I knew why I had screamed in nameless terror when Dr. M had asked me to fantasy the act of masturbation. That nameless terror was now named: it was the dreadful punishment of being confined in a strait jacket, were I to "play with myself."

Now I knew why I had been suffering those terrible tensions in my arms. Those tensions were an unconscious reminder of the great struggle I had had, as a two-year-old, to free my arms from the strait jacket. No wonder those tensions had returned in my later life, during periods of stress; they were the conditioned behavioral response of my earliest stress, which had been too great to overcome.

This was the reconstruction I made that night, as I lay awake. Fantastic, marvelous. Even as I marveled, though, I was struck with a new puzzlement: what had these things to do with the chief problem of the session—the enema dilemma??

Here I stopped, with a chuckle at my insatiability. In a little over two months of LSD therapy, I had been cured of lifelong frigidity. There would be lots of time to worry through this enema business, whatever it was. In fact, there was to be another session in three days' time. With that attractive view in prospect, I fell asleep and slept the deep untroubled sleep of a baby—or rather, the deep sleep of an untroubled baby.

Three days later, when I went for my eleventh session, I reported triumphantly to Dr. E my series of discoveries: the existence of a real Miss Leahy; the existence of two real itching rashes, chicken pox and measles; which had probably caused me to scratch at myself, to discover masturbation, and to have been "punished" by having my arms pinned into a strait jacket (rather than being prevented from scarring myself) . . . all of which explained my unconscious terror of masturbation.

But I still did not know how the enema nozzle fitted into this scene.

"Why not try the enema fantasy again, and see if you can find out?"

I dreaded going back to those insanely cruel tortures which the enema fantasy had produced in the last session—but back I went.

Once again the nozzle penetrated me and changed into a red-hot poker into an acetylene blowtorch back to a nozzle into a steel drill into a blowtorch. Miss Leahy kept changing, too: into my father, into a devil, into Dr. M, into William, even into Arthur, the man with whom I had had my first unrequited love affair. All the while the pain being inflicted on me increased to what should have been an unendurable level, but it was not unendurable because it remained and remained without ever reaching a climax. Worse. At times I felt pleasure in the very pain—and hated myself for feeling it. However, those pleasurable moments were extremely brief and converted right back into torture. At length I rebelled. I refused to suffer these tortures any more.

Dr. E interposed then to explain that such physical (or psychical) "pleasure in pain" is the classic reaction of the masochist; and that masochism was the specific problem I was facing in the session. I freely granted my psychical masochism. Indeed, I had explored it lengthily and fruitlessly in psychoanalysis. In all of my relationships with men, with the exception of my husband by some miraculous good fortune, I had invariably chosen to love some man who would not return my love. This pattern had existed from earliest high school crushes to my most recent involvement with William—and the current absurd but real love, unobtainable Dr. M. Each and every time I would cling to an unrequited love, which would give me the "pleasure" of being rejected. Again and again and again. I added gloomily that this monotonous pattern of behavior was so deep-rooted that I would never be able to change it. . . .

Dr. E contradicted me. One of the purposes of psychotherapy, he said, was to find the reason behind a neurotic behavior pattern such as this "need" of mine to be rejected. Often the "need" is based on a misconception stemming from one's formative years. If I could unearth that misconception from my unconscious, probably my drive to be rejected would disappear—or be replaced by the more healthy drive of finding someone to love who would return my love.

This was a prospect infinitely pleasing: how to achieve it? Dr. E recommended as a start that I fantasy the enema again—this time, trying to go beyond the static level of pain, through to its climax. I realized then that I had been stopping at an *unfulfilled* level of pain, just as I had always stopped in sex at an *unfulfilled* level of pleasure.

All right. I would try to let the pain consume me . . . and see what the climax would be.

I began with the simple fantasy of Miss Leahy giving me an enema. Again the nozzle transformed into a red-hot poker, a steel drill, a nozzle, a blowtorch. Maelstrom of torture, but I was never consumed in it.

At length I cleared away the maelstrom and returned to the basic fantasy of Miss Leahy giving me, a two-year-old baby, an enema. The water poured into me, hot hot water relentlessly poured into me. I felt a swift cramping pain, surging stronger and stronger until I could only writhe and scream uncontrollably, until I felt myself exploding into thousands of scattered pieces. . . .

I lay dazed, shattered, unable to move or feel or think. After a time I heard Dr. E repeat a question he had been asking which I had not understood:

"What happened to you?"

"I . . . I don't know. I just . . . exploded . . . burst. That's all."

As the tiny pieces of me began to coalesce, I felt outrage: What the HELL had been the purpose behind all that?? What possible therapeutic value could this self-inflicted torture produce? How DARE Dr. E subject ANYONE to such an experience?? Even as I unleashed this fury, a new fantasy emerged:

My brother, with demonic fury, was pulling the breasts off my body. I struggled to stop him but he overpowered me and tore them completely off. They clung to his fingers like taffy. He ate the taffy, then licked his fingers clean.

I felt desolated. Now I could never become a woman. Ever. What could I do . . . ?

"Why don't you get your breasts back again?"

"*How?*"

"How do *you* think?"

The only answer that occurred to me was to go down into my brother's stomach to get back the taffy which had been my breasts. I did that in fantasy—but then I could not find my way out. I began walking through the long dark tunnel of his intestines . . . until . . . at the far end of the tunnel . . . I saw a light . . . and I walked toward the light . . . but then the light disappeared. . . . My brother had closed the exit . . . I was trapped . . . worse. . . . I saw that he had closed up the exit with the enema nozzle . . . he was going to drown me in the water that was pouring out of it. . . . I was going to be drowned in this tunnel where there was no escape. . . .

Panic—until I realized I did not have to drown. All I need do was turn the enema nozzle into my brother! Immediately in fantasy I did exactly that. . . .

And with the conscious part of me, I realized I had reversed roles: *I* was now the one inflicting torture rather than the one *being* tortured. I was the sadist instead of the masochist. But that was just as bad. I did not want to be sadist *or* masochist—

Dr. E recommended that I stop intellectualizing, and continue the fantasy.

Back to the enema nozzle and my brother. I kept pouring the water into him . . . and his body swelled larger and larger . . . until *he* became a giant balloon of a body . . . until *he* screamed and screamed as he burst into thousands of pieces. I found myself in the middle of his scream.

"I'm a scream." I heard myself say with a giggle. "Have you ever been a scream, doctor? I'm a long scream through a tunnel———"

Conscious Me gasped.

How many times during these last weeks had that sentence come all unbidden into my head? "I'm a long scream through a tunnel." When had I first said it? Wasn't it with Dr. M? Yes. . . . When I had wrapped my arms around my body (in just the position Miss Leahy had pinned my arms in the strait jacket) and had said: "I feel as if I were going to burst or explode." And then I had added: "I'm a long scream through the tunnel."

Those two sentences had recurred again and again to puzzle me. In a session with Dr. M I had fantasied "going through the tunnel" many times, without learning what the tunnel was. Or the scream. Or the explosion. I had not found out about them until this moment here and now:

Presumably sometime during the summer when I had been ill with the itching rashes of chicken pox and measles, Miss Leahy had given me an enema, which had been too hot and too strong. As the water poured into my baby body, I must have felt that I was going to "burst or explode." I must have screamed with the pain: or else the pain had shot through my intestines like "a long scream through the tunnel."

Enema nozzle.

"I feel as if I were going to burst or explode."

"I'm a long scream through the tunnel."

Itching rash. Masturbation. Arm tensions. Yes yes yes, every one of these symptoms seemed related to that summer when I was two and a half years old, ill with chicken pox and measles; when I had been pinned down in a strait jacket and given an enema.

These were the nuclei of my neurosis: strait jacket and enema nozzle. The strait jacket had taught me that feeling pleasure "down there" led to punishment and pain. That lesson was drilled home by the enema nozzle: any instrument going in to me down there would prove so painful that I would explode into a long scream through the tunnel.

Sudden question: Could I have confused an enema nozzle inserted into the anus with a penis inserted into the vagina? I answered the question for myself with an emphatic yes. As a baby, I probably had had no notion of the differences between the vagina, urethra, and anus. As a matter of fact, in these enema fantasies, I had seen myself attacked *in all three apertures at the same time.* Furthermore, I had seen the enema nozzle change into a buzz saw and a steel drill—just as in earlier sex fantasies I had seen the penis change into a buzz saw and steel drill (among other things).

Yes. Unconsciously I had equated the enema nozzle with the penis: both were instruments of torture which would, if I were to feel anything, explode me into a long scream through the tunnel.

At long long last, I had uncovered the classic Freudian "trauma" responsible for my sexual difficulty: one too-strong, too-hot enema, received when I was two and a half years old.[3] It was preposterous. But undeniable. . . .

I lay on the couch, feeling absolutely marvelous. I had been categorically cured. I was now a whole and wholesome woman.

"Isn't it marvelous?" I said. "I've been cured."

Once again, this revelation burst upon me in a moment of time. But I want to emphasize that I could not articulate what had happened. I could not itemize the symptoms, nor the causes of them. I only felt the bell of truth ring in me, when I recognized the trauma.

Later in the week I was to wonder whether the symptoms which had been plaguing me would disappear, now that I had resolved the enema dilemma and had found out the reasons for my peculiar complaints.

As a matter of record, all symptoms disappeared. I was never again troubled by an itching rash, the enema nozzle or blowtorch or steel drill or buzz saw or red-hot poker, I never again felt I was a "long scream through the tunnel," nor did I feel that I was about to burst or explode—not under the drug, nor in life.

14.

Celle Qui Fût la Belle Heaulmière

WE WERE still in the eleventh session.

"Isn't it marvelous? I'm cured," I repeated, because Dr. E had not answered me. I wanted him to say that he too was pleased with my cure. Instead, he asked an idiotic question:

"What happened to your breasts?"

"*What!*"

"In that last fantasy, you went inside your brother to get your breasts back. What happened to them?"

"Oh for God's sake—!" Much disgust. "I have them now. I'm a full-grown, normal, healthy woman."

"Well . . . we've still some time left. How about showing yourself to your father as a normal, healthy woman?"

"If you think it's necessary." I was annoyed. Apparently Dr. E did not think I was cured at all. Well, I would prove it. I would in fantasy present myself to my father as a healthy and normal woman.

When I did—strange things happened:

My breasts began to dwindle, and I began to grow smaller. My breasts and I kept right on growing smaller and smaller, until I became a little flat-chested girl who was clinging to her father's hand.

Disconcertment. I was *not* that dependent little girl clinging to her father. Not any more. I was *not*. And I would prove it. I would repeat the fantasy, and this time I would *remain a woman*.

I did repeat the fantasy, and I remained a woman . . . but then my father began to change. He grew larger . . . more powerful. . . much more powerful . . . in fact . . . he transformed into a huge gorilla. The gorilla began chasing me through a forest. I fled as fast as I could because I knew that if the gorilla were to catch me, he would destroy me.

Faster and faster I ran . . . but not fast enough . . . because now the gorilla had caught me . . . one of his huge paws was around my throat . . . he was choking me.

Struggle to break free. Violent, useless struggle because the gorilla was too powerful. I was choking to death. Suffocating, gasping at words, trying desperately to explain what was happening. But I could only make stuttering, gasping sounds because the gorilla was choking me so tightly. I had no words, no words at all . . .

"Oh, for God's sake!"

Conscious Me had spoken in a loud clear voice and had broken the fantasy.

I found myself backed halfway up a wall, gripping my throat with one of my hands, so tightly that I had been able to make only spluttering noises.

Discovery: All these weeks I had been suffering with stuttering and mutism—I had probably been expressing this unconscious fear of being *choked* by Gorilla-Father. Obviously, he was still a threat. In spite of my "cure."

But I believed I really *was* cured. This fantasy of a gorilla choking me had just been a last ditch stand of my masochism. But I was not going to be a masochist any more. Nor was I going to be a little girl any more. Nor was I going to be dependent on father any more. I was determined to be rid of all that nonsense.

For a third time I presented myself to father as a normal,

healthy woman. In this fantasy, neither my father nor I underwent any metamorphosis. I told my father that I was a mature woman who could enjoy sex fully without any fear of being destroyed or hurt by it. My father listened attentively, and accepted what I told him.

"There!" Exultantly. "I told you I was cured!"

"Fine," Dr. E answered. "Why don't you fantasy a *good* sex experience now—with anyone you like?"

Here was a bountiful gift from Dr. E. No more Oedipus!

I promptly chose for my partner—Dr. M. (Incredibly, I still believed I was in love with him.) Now: to have a *good* experience of sex.

Oddly, although I had chosen my One True Love for this fantasy, I was extremely reluctant to begin it. It suddenly seemed all wrong to be indulging in sex before a third person. In fact, it was a degenerate thing to be asked to do. Dr. E was no better than a Peeping Tom. He wanted me to do a disgusting and degrading——

Conscious Me began to giggle. For several weeks I had been exhibiting myself to this Peeping Tom in a most intimate assortment of sexual studies. Why should I feel embarrassed at *this* stage of therapy? Dr. E turned the question right back to me. I heard myself say that perhaps my embarrassment was another resistance: perhaps I was still afraid of being mutilated and destroyed in the act of sex.

"Good sex feelings are mighty hard to come by," Dr. E concurred.

Challenge. Good sex feelings certainly *had* been hard for me to come by. But I could have them now. And I would.

As background for the fantasy of Dr. M and myself, I chose a beautiful, deep-green forest glade—which, to my intense chagrin, became the same forest where the gorilla had choked me to death.

Hell and damnation. In spite of my insistence that I was genuinely in love with Dr. M, that he did *not* represent the

Omnipotent Sadist, I had just put him in fantasy where the Omnipotent Gorilla had been.

I was very angry, now. I categorically refused to believe that I was incapable of good sex feelings. I would start this fantasy again (*not* in that damned forest), and I would carry it through to ecstasy.

But I was so overcome with shyness and embarrassment again that I could not even begin.

"Why can't you?"

"Well . . . because . . ."

"Because what?"

(Sometimes I hated that inexorable curiosity in Dr. E.)

"Well . . . because . . . because . . . it isn't real. I mean . . . well . . . Dr. M isn't in love with me."

"He could be, for the purpose of fantasy. Anything is possible in fantasy."

That was true. I had fantasied all sorts of impossible events under LSD: from being exploded by a Purple Screw, to being set on fire with acetylene blowtorches, to eating thousands of hard-boiled eggs through a desert. All of these fantasies had been extremely *painful*, in reality. It was time to stop that masochistic nonsense. It was time to fantasy a *pleasurable* experience. Yes, I would fantasy that Dr. M loved me just as much as I loved him, and we would consummate our love.

Not for one moment could I imagine that Dr. M was in love with me. He could never be in love with me. For that matter, no man could. I was an impossible object for physical love. In fact, I had become in fantasy *Celle Qui Fût la Belle Heaulmière*, that remarkable Rodin sculpture of a scrawny hag with withered dugs.

Why should I see myself as Heaulmière? I did not have a body like hers. I was no longer an Ugly Duckling. I was regularly invited out to dinner by one or another man these days. That was the *reality*. And since it was the reality, I refused to see myself as Heaulmière. I would create instead an image of myself as I look today.

I could not. I literally could not. I remained Heaulmière, to the very end of the session. . . .

Clearly, I had uncovered another psychic reality which would have to be dissipated before I could arrive at good sex feelings. I would have to see myself as a woman attractive enough to be loved before I could enjoy the experience of love. And I *would*.

In spite of this setback, I left Dr. E's office in a haze of delight. After all, I had unearthed the infantile trauma which had been a basic cause of my frigidity. That I was still unable to surrender to good sex-and-love feelings was a minor problem, which I should be able to resolve in the next sessions.

One or two nights later, as I was driving home and thinking of the many tortures and terrors I had endured under LSD, I congratulated myself: it seemed that I was very nearly finished with therapy for there was just about nothing left to fear.

As if on cue, I saw an image of someone coming at me as if to choke me—and I was promptly terrified. Fortunately for the other cars on the road my fright was superseded by wonder: why should I have felt such terror at the thought of someone choking me? No one had ever tried to choke me, so far as I knew. And thinking consciously now of someone choking me did not frighten me in the least. I determined in the next session to explore this unexpected, irrational fear.

With the typical perversity of my conscious mind I forgot all about the incident. Perhaps because, in the days that followed, I suffered two or three rejections which, although admittedly minor rejections, nevertheless made me feel like the Ugly Heaulmière whom no one could possibly love. One of these rejections I should like to describe:

The most recent of my Unrequited Loves, William, arrived in town on one of his rare visits and telephoned me. Since I had decided to end our masochistic "love" affair and had stopped corresponding with him several weeks before, his phone call took me by surprise. As he talked with me, I felt a strong desire to see him—a desire I resented and pushed aside. And when

William in his oblique way implied that he would like to see me, I ignored the overture. He rang off without making a date with me. Whereupon I was swamped in depression. I had been rejected again.

Or had I? Had William rejected me, or had I brought the rejection on myself just so that I could have the dubious delight of this rejection-and-depression blues called masochism?? After all, I myself had decided not to write to him or to see him any more . . . but on the other hand . . . I *did* want to see him. . . .

I knew this conflict of opposing emotions very well. I even knew the technical word for it. Ambivalence. Whatever the word, I hated being back in the dreary pattern of finding some-one to punish me (even courting the punishment this time, by ignoring William's indirect invitation on the telephone) and then feeling unloved, unwanted, and all the rest of it. Did I really seek out rejection-and-depression blues? I determined to find out, next session.

As usual, the night before the session, I was sleepless until six in the morning. About four o'clock, just as I was falling asleep, a fleeting dream or fantasy frightened me awake:

I had been seated next to Dr. M, who was driving a car. As he drove, he made a strange gesture with his thumb and forefinger, pressing two instruments on the dashboard of the car. That was the entire image.

But it had jarred me awake, and left me with a heart pounding heavily in fear, real fear. Why was I so afraid?

I tried to find out why by recreating the picture of Dr. M making that peculiar gesture with his thumb and forefinger on two instruments of a dashboard.

Gradually the gesture and the dashboard began to look familiar. Then I remembered. When I was a little girl, the family had owned a car with a dashboard like that, and my father had occasionally made that gesture with his thumb and forefinger on those two instruments. But his gesture had never frightened me as a child. Why did it now?

I looked carefully with my mind's eyes at the twin instruments on the dashboard, hoping they would furnish a clue. They were unfamiliar instruments . . . obsolete now . . . what had they been . . . ? In the next instant I recognized them. One had been labeled THROTTLE and the other CHOKE.

Another chill of fear before I understood: this had been another choke-image.

Two weeks ago I had been frightened awake by a dream or fantasy of my brother coming at me, as if to *choke* me. In the last session I had been violently *choked* by a huge gorilla who had metamorphosed out of my father. Now Dr. M had made a gesture on the *choke* and *throttle,* while he was driving a car. This last thought brought back the memory of the incident I had forgotten during the week: that when I had been driving a car, congratulating myself that I had nothing left to fear—I had been suddenly terrified by an image of someone coming at me, to *choke* me. What was all this *choke* business??

An odd association popped into my mind. For several years— at rare times—I would be on the verge of falling asleep, only to be jarred awake by a constriction in my throat which made me cough. As a result, I always kept some water on the bedtable, to smooth over the constriction should it occur.

I sat up in bed and drank some of the water and wondered whether that strange constriction in my throat could be connected to these choke-images—and if so, how? No answer came. But these choke-symbols seemed a good gambit with which to start the next day's session.

15.

The "Ticking"

AFTER taking the pills for the twelfth session, I began to puzzle over the previous night's image of Dr. M's fingers on the THROTTLE and CHOKE . . . and was suddenly startled by the eruption of an old, odd physical symptom. Now it is time to describe it and give its history.

Some ten years before I began LSD therapy, I took a course in relaxation. The course was deeply interesting because I discovered that I could *not* relax until I learned to release certain tensions—*of which I had been totally unaware.* One of these hitherto unconscious tensions, located in my neck and throat, proved more obstinate than any of the others. When I first grew aware of it, I was startled by its strength: it was as if something were gripping my neck and throat in a vise. The more I tried to release the tension, the more persistently it gripped me. I battled it for weeks, until one fine day in class I felt it dissolve. As it did, I heard a most strange "clicking" or "ticking" sound coming out of my neck and throat. This was *not* an imagined clicking or ticking. It was a real sound, loud enough to disturb the other students in class who asked me to stop making that noise. But I could not. It was being produced quite independently of my will. After a few minutes, the ticking stopped —again, independently.

In the years which followed, at strange times and places, the clicking noise would erupt and taunt me. On the bus, in an office, at the theater. Some six months after it began, I went to the family doctor. Not because the ticking was painful (it was not in the least) but because it was disconcerting, downright embarrassing, to have strangers stare at me as if I were possessed of a time bomb. I proceeded to click for the doctor (by this time I could produce the sound at will although I could not always stop it at will), who listened with some incredulity. Then he examined my neck and throat and several other places too. Finally he announced that he could find no organic reason for my affliction and advised me, since it was not painful, to ignore it. This was a piece of advice I found difficult to follow.

"She's ticking again!" became a familiar jibe as, year after year at odd intervals, the clicking would involuntarily begin. I was still clicking when I began LSD therapy. In fact, I had ticked occasionally during a session, but I had never been able to associate any thought or image or emotion to the symptom—except once in an early session with Dr. M, when I had been reminded of an episode that had taken place an evening or two before the session:

I had been at a dinner party and had made an unusually bad pun. In retaliation, one of the guests had come toward me with his arms outstretched as if to choke me. I began to laugh, but then felt an uprush of fear as his hands approached my throat. My fear was so obvious that the gentleman stopped "choking" me. Some two or three minutes later the ticking began—so loudly that the guest (seated at least four feet from me now) asked what that ticking noise was, and was it perhaps coming from a clock he did not see?

(I want to emphasize that this episode occurred some two months previously, in an early session with Dr. M. It had seemed irrelevant then, and I had dismissed it. Actually it was not until I was collating all of the reports, in preparing for this book, that I rediscovered the incident and realized it was the very first of these frightening choke images. Someone at a dinner party coming at me as if to choke me had elicited the same unreasonable fear that I had experienced when, driving home, I had seemed to see someone coming to choke me; when just as I was falling asleep I had seen a dream or fantasy of my brother coming at me as if to choke me; when under LSD I had been pursued and choked by the gorilla which had metamorphosed out of my father; and when, again as I was falling asleep, I had seen in dream or fantasy an image of Dr. M making a gesture on the throttle and choke.)

None of these similarities occurred to me at the beginning of this twelfth session, when the ticking in my throat erupted. Instead, as the ticking grew louder and louder, I began to panic. Then Dr. E appeared.

"Do you hear *that?* It sounds as if—as if I'd swallowed a clock!"

I had not known I was going to say those words, and when I heard them I began to laugh as if I had made an extravagantly funny joke. That dispelled my panic, and I explained to Dr. E how the image of Dr. M's fingers on the CHOKE and THROTTLE had seemed to bring on the clicking, which was still going on at a noisy rate. Dr. E suggested I explore Dr. M's gesture in a fantasy.

Here began an indiscriminate barrage of fantasies, all of which seemed meaningless. In retrospect, I was able to isolate three fragments which are worth reporting. *But only in retrospect.*

In the middle of something or other, for no apparent reason, I suddenly saw myself as a small child curled around my father in bed. This image became vivid, and remained. Then I realized that this was not a fantasy at all; but rather a remembrance (or reliving?) of a minor and forgotten episode from childhood. When I was perhaps four or five years old, I had gone into my parents' bedroom one Sunday morning, and had wakened father. Since he wanted to go on sleeping, he suggested I get into bed too. It was a rare treat to get into my parents' big bed. I climbed up into it happily, and curled around my father's back. I did not expect to sleep. I never went back to sleep once

I was awake. But this time, unprecedentedly, I did fall asleep.
And was wakened by mother *at ten o'clock!* Surprise and delight. I had never slept so late before. Only grownups slept so
late. . . . As I recited this mild bit of remembrance, I felt the
shock of realization.

My usual waking hour in adult life has always been *ten
o'clock.* I had supposed that I woke at that late hour because
as an actress I had worked in theaters late into the night. But
now that rationalization did not seem right . . . after all . . .
I had not acted in the theater for several years. . . .

Oedipus? I did not pursue the question but rushed on to
other fantasies.

Some time later, I found myself again curled around my
father as he lay sleeping in bed. This time I was not a child, but
a baby. In the brief moment this image lasted, I saw that my
father's body was blue and mine was red. Blue father. Red me.
Incomprehensible image.

(It was not until much later that this image became compre-
hensible. Unpleasantly so. I had seen my father as blue, me as
red. One or another combination of *red and blue* (purple, violet, amethyst) had consistently colored the threatening images
of LSD: Purple Screw, Purplish Peapod, Amethyst Necklace,
Inviolate/In Violet, Purplish Foetus, etc., etc. Could this color
threat be the symbolic blending of father's blue body and my
red one? Oedipus again?)

The third fragment proved of major importance—but again
only in retrospect. At the time it seemed just as irrelevant as the
rest of the afternoon's material. Moreover: it was *contrived,*
deliberately, toward the end of the session when the drug no
longer seemed to be working. At that juncture I complained
that the last few fantasies seemed to be the result of a remark
my mother had made about the measles-and-chicken-pox summer with Miss Leahy, to the effect that until my sister was born,
I had always slept in a crib in my parents' bedroom.

After registering this complaint, I wondered aloud whether
I might have seen anything of a sexual nature in that room—

which event, if it had occurred, would fit right into the classic Freudian concept of the "primal scene": a very small child or baby observing parental intercourse. Dr. E suggested I fantasy such a scene. I agreed, but stated categorically that I remembered *nothing* of sleeping in my parents' bedroom when I was a baby and that whatever I fantasied would be pure invention.

Immediately and effortlessly, an invention: I was a baby, standing in my crib, looking over to my parents' bed . . . where they were . . . what? . . . so strange . . . they were . . . all wrapped around each other . . . and my father was doing . . . what was he doing? . . . something . . . something terrible . . . like he was . . . he was choking my mother . . . choking her . . . I felt sick all of a sudden. So sick . . . to think how he must be hurting mother . . . but mother just let him choke her . . . and after a little while they both sort of smiled . . . and turned over and went to sleep . . . and then . . . I moved to the back of my crib . . . and I scratched my nearly hairless head . . . and said:

"Well . . . I just won't feel anything and then it won't hurt."

I was almost unaware that I had spoken those words. When I heard them, I gasped.

"I just won't feel anything and then it won't hurt."

In still another context, in still another situation, I had expressed the old neurotic fear of being *hurt* in the act of sex. The same neurotic fear I had already expressed in fantasies of the Purple Screw, the Purplish Poisonous Peapod, the enema, the strait jacket, the electrical blowtorch, the steel drill, etc., etc. How many factors could there be for my frigidity? I was to learn much later that almost every neurotic symptom (such as this of frigidity) is the result of *many* factors.[1]

This resurgence of the frigidity motif totally obscured for me the more pertinent meaning of this fantasy. To wit: I had uncovered the original frightening choke-image. I had seen, as a baby in a crib, how my father "choked" my mother.

(Whether I really did see this happen when I was a baby in a crib, or whether this was only a fantasy *invented* under LSD, belongs again to the problem of reality versus psychic reality.)

To repeat: I was not aware of having made this discovery— or *any* discovery—that afternoon. I left Dr. E, disconsolate at the barrenness of the session. I had not learned why I had ticked nor why I was so afraid of being choked.

In spite of the barren session, I woke the next morning, feeling splendid. Incredibly, I had quite forgotten the depression I had been suffering. Even more incredibly, I had forgotten all about the choke-images. (In the terminology, I had *re-repressed* these symptoms.)

This feeling of well-being continued throughout the week, so that again I believed that I was nearly cured. All I need do was rid my psyche of Ugly Heaulmière so that I would feel capable of being loved; of enjoying fully the pleasures of sex.

It was with pleasant anticipation, then, that I stayed at home the night before the next session, reading and—just before turning out the light to sleep—leafing through the book of Rodin sculptures. No full bladder appeared to send me up and off to the bathroom. No fleeting impressions came to frighten me awake. I fell asleep promptly, slept deeply, woke refreshed, and went off to the doctor in a state of elation.

Having utterly "forgotten" those rejection-and-depression blues, and the choke-images, I was thoroughly disconcerted, in the half-hour preceding the thirteenth session, by another violent eruption of the ticking in my neck and throat. After the initial shock, I determined not to panic but to "go with the ticking" and see what image would come.

No image did come. Instead I remembered how in the last session I had cried that "I had swallowed a clock!" and then had laughed at my joke.

Now the joke did not seem a joke at all. Because I suddenly remembered that *for many years I had not been able to sleep in a room where a clock ticked, even softly.*

Perhaps—figuratively—I *had* swallowed a clock? Perhaps . . . I should fantasy what kind of clock I had swallowed?

I relaxed as much as I could with the ticking so loud in my ears . . . and I seemed to see . . . hazily . . . an old-fashioned clock. Just then, Dr. E joined me. I told him what I was trying to do and he suggested I continue.

Again I tried to fantasy the clock I had swallowed which was ticking now so loudly in my throat. Again I saw a hazy old-fashioned clock . . . which as I watched it . . . became more clearly etched. It was a kitchen alarm clock with an aluminum alarm bell on its top, a black dial with luminous green numbers.

But the buzzing black came rushing up to drown out the image. I forced myself to plunge through the buzzing black, back to the old-fashioned kitchen clock. When I managed to see it clearly again, the luminous green numerals on its black face began to emit a vaporous gas which was going to anesthetize me. I fought off this second resistance, and recreated the image of the clock.

This time—nothing happened at all. The clock simply remained an old-fashioned black-dialed kitchen alarm clock. I did not recognize it. I did not remember ever having owned a clock like that. I did not remember ever having seen a clock like that. Ever. Why should I have conjured up this particular clock?

Dr. E recommended that I keep watching the clock, that perhaps it would change into something that I would recognize.

It did not. I kept staring at the clock but it remained, obstinately, an unfamiliar kitchen alarm clock. At length—to my conscious surprise—I heard myself speak in the voice of a very small child:

"I've got to keep looking at the clock."

"Why?"

"Well . . . if I keep looking at it . . ." My voice sounded younger still. ". . . then . . . then . . . I won't be able to . . . look . . . at the bed."

"What bed?"

"Where Mommy and Daddy are."

"Maybe you'd better look over there."

Wild fear in me, the wild fear of a baby.

Yes, I had become a baby now . . . whimpering . . . and . . . I was standing in a crib . . . staring at a black-dialed clock . . . and I had to keep staring at it . . . because it would be terrible to look over to the bed. . . .

Conscious Me heard Dr. E say that I should look away from the clock to the bed but Baby Me was so afraid, so very afraid.

Long long struggle. Finally . . . Baby Me managed to look away from the clock . . . past the rim of the crib . . . over to the bed where . . . my father and mother were . . . quietly sleeping.

Why had I been so afraid to look? I was not at all afraid any more. In fact, I got out of the crib and into bed between my father and mother. Then my father woke up and was angry to find me there. He complained to my mother that I was always getting into bed with them. That made me feel bad. I had done something bad again. I was always doing something bad and my father was always getting angry with me. I kept on feeling bad, while my mother took me out of their bed and put me back in the crib.

There the fantasy ended. Which was disappointing because the clock was still ticking in my throat. How could I stop it?

Dr. E suggested I repeat the fantasy.

Back I went into the crib, where I kept staring at the clock so that I would not be able to look over to the bed. Another struggle to overcome the fear. When I managed to look away from the clock, past the rim of the crib, over to the bed . . . I saw something . . . something so peculiar . . . lying between my parents . . . what was it? . . . weird and and and . . .

I felt badly confused suddenly and stopped talking.

"What did you see?" Dr. E prodded me.

"I don't really know." It was hard to find words. "It was

. . . well . . . sort of . . . well . . . brown fluff . . . like when you sweep up a room . . . sort of furry brown fluff . . ."

"What does the fluff make you think of?"

"Nothing. Except . . . but that's silly."

"Say it anyhow."

The furry fluff had made me think of a story I had read long ago. Although I could not remember the name of the story or its author (nor have I been able to locate either one since), I did remember the plot:

It was about a man who one day did something evil. When he returned to his room, he found a small piece of brown fluff on the floor which was difficult to get rid of. As the story developed, the man perpetrated more and more evil. After each new exploit the fluff would reappear in his room, larger and more clinging. Then: the man committed murder. He dreaded returning to his room for fear of the furry brown thing which had by now become menacing. When he did return to his room, he was relieved to find it empty of the fur thing, and he quickly locked his door. Shortly afterwards, the door flung itself open. Leaning against it, huge, upright, without head or tail, boa-like, was the Fur Thing—which enveloped the man and crushed him to death.

That was the story. Why had I remembered it *now??*

Stupid. Except—

I was that furry fluff in bed between my father and mother. What was I doing there? Why was I the Fur Thing? Dr. E suggested I continue the fantasy. I understood none of it but decided to go on being the Fur Thing in bed between my parents. For a while nothing happened. But then my parents wanted to make love. I did not want them to. It was easy to prevent them. All I had to do, as the Fur Thing, was to roll myself into a soft brown ball and go inside Mother. That would keep Father from penetrating into her. I was in my mother now as the Fur Thing . . . and I began to grow larger and larger . . . until I realized I had changed into a human embryo with a monstrously large head . . . an embryo in its

fourth month . . . and as that four-month-old embryo the
fantasy came to an end.

What the devil had all that been about?

Dr. E recommended I repeat the fantasy. I was willing—but
not as that Evil Fur Thing. I put myself back into the crib as
a baby and began to watch the clock all over again. This time
it was not too difficult to look away from the clock and over to
the bed . . . but as I did . . . I heard myself begin to cry
. . . loudly . . . because I wanted to be in bed with my
parents but they did not want me to be in bed with them . . .
so I kept on crying . . . and then I began to feel that dreadful
full bladder (for the first time in weeks) . . . and its pressure
grew stronger . . . much much stronger . . . and finally, after
so much frustration . . . finally . . . I wet the bed in fantasy.
I was sitting in the wet cold sheets of the crib and I was crying
very loudly because it felt so awful and I felt so awful because
I knew I had done that bad thing again and I knew I would
go right on doing that same bad thing so long as my father and
mother kept me in their bedroom but not in their bed with
them. I realized, then, that they *had* put me out of their room
and into a bedroom with my brother, but there too I kept
wetting the bed because I wanted to be back in my parents'
bedroom and in bed with them.

That was why I had been a chronic bed-wetter!

This discovery ended the fantasy—and created instead frustration—and fury. My badness and my bed-wetting had been
the *reality*. Not the psychic reality but the *reality*. But what
good did it do to know all this?

"OK! I used to wet the bed because I wanted to be in bed
with my father and mother. But how the *hell* does that solve
anything? My father and mother were right to keep me out of
their bed and I was wrong to want to get into their bed but
what the HELL does that fact have to do with the ticking in
my throat?"

This, considerably expurgated, was the nature of my complaint to Dr. E, who merely suggested that I repeat the fantasy
of getting into bed with my parents.

I rebelled. I had done this idiotic clock fantasy several times now and nothing out of all the stuff I had conjured up had anything to do with ANYTHING much less the ticking in my throat etc. etc.

Eventually I gave up the rebellion and returned to the same bedroom, same crib, same clock, same parents in their bed. Suddenly I was the same Fur Thing in bed between my parents. I did not want to be that Evil Fur Thing *at all*. But try as I would, I could not put myself back in the crib as a baby. Somehow though, still lying between my parents, I changed from the Evil Fur Thing into a baby . . . who began to grow smaller . . . much much smaller . . . so miniscule now that my parents did not even know I was in bed with them . . . and then they began to make love. I found myself, a tiny creature, straddled across their united parts . . . feeling their pleasure . . . their pleasure*s* . . . yes, it was as if I were *both* my father's sex and my mother's sex, wondrous sensation . . . *but why should I be feeling both pleasures?*

Dr. E recommended that I not stop to question anything but simply *feel*.

I did . . . and found that this remarkable twin pleasure expanded into the ecstasy of an orgasm which continued on and on and on and on, and as it did the fantasy changed.

I became a nude woman sprawled against the sky . . . and I was no longer ashamed of my body . . . quite the reverse . . . I felt the beauty in me and in sex and in love . . . and now I was with Dr. M who loved me as much as I loved him.

Shock of wonder and delight. I was no longer Ugly Heaulmière. She had disappeared and in her place had come beauty and love and ecstasy.

Through the ecstasy Dr. M and I submerged into the sparkling black which was no longer buzzing, no longer frightening, but part of the ecstasy.

In this sparkling black we transformed into one Rodin sculpture after another. Now we were The Kiss . . . and then *L'Emprise* . . . *L'Emprise* which was no longer painful or cruel but ecstatic, yes, it was ecstatic to be the woman pierced through by the man in an act of love . . . and now we were the Mary Magdalene embracing the crucified Jesus as if the heat of her body and sex could bring him back to life . . . and now we became Les Oceanides, two creatures dissolving into a cosmos of rock at the climax of their love.

Then the Rodin sculptures disappeared.

And I became Rodin himself, who knew that sex encompassed all delight and all perversion, all good and all evil: simultaneously I felt the pleasure of a man's body and the pain of being pierced by a red-hot poker and the distress of a full bladder and the merging into cosmos and all this was a part of sex which comprises good and evil intermingled and I was large enough now to encompass this knowledge and ecstasy which remained and remained——

Without the climactic moment of release.

From very far away, I heard Dr. E propose a five-minute rest.

I lay transfigured. For the second time in my life I had achieved an orgasm of monumental physical pleasure.

Gradually it occurred to me that on both occasions I had not felt the ultimate moment of release . . . why had I not felt that shattering moment? . . . the transcendent afterglow bathed me and prevented me from thinking any more. . . .

Eventually Dr. E asked me where I was. I managed to focus back to the present moment and the puzzle I had come upon: why did I never feel the ultimate moment? I felt ridiculous for asking the question. Suspension in orgasm was the most exquisite sensation I had ever known, and yet I was dissatisfied. . . .

Dr. E did not seem to resent my dissatisfaction. In fact, he suggested I might have still another block which we had not yet explored.

I was willing to make the exploration but had no idea where to begin. Besides, I heard myself protesting, I did not *want* another sexual fantasy so soon again. I could not possibly achieve that level of ecstasy—nor should I. It would be indulgence. I had come here today to solve a specific problem and it was time to return to it. For several moments I could not even think what the specific problem was. But then I remembered: of course, it was that silly ticking in my throat. I had been trying to find out what that ticking clock I had "swallowed" was meant to symbolize. I heard myself propose that I repeat the clock fantasy. (This proposal astonished Conscious Me, who had just a little while ago rebelled at the "idiotic" fantasy.)

Once more I became a baby in a crib, watching the black-dialed kitchen clock, hoping this time it would change into the thing it symbolized. It did not. It remained, infuriatingly, an old-fashioned Alarm Clock.

When at length I looked away from the clock over to my parents' bed, I saw that they were making love. The Alarm Clock began to ring its bell loudly, as if its ringing could stop their lovemaking. But it did not. I heard myself ask what else the Alarm Clock could do to stop them? I was amazed at the answer I gave myself, which was that the clock could become a time bomb . . . and then it did become a time bomb . . . and now it was inside my mother . . . and I was counting down to zero . . . and at zero the bomb exploded, annihilating my mother.

"I'm glad! Even though the clock had to be smashed too!— NO! This is *my* fantasy! The clock doesn't have to be destroyed!"

Horror at these words in Conscious Me but there was no time for horror because the Alarm Clock was intact again, but so was my mother, and she was furious. She picked up the Alarm Clock and hurled it against a wall, smashing it into bits.

"NO! She *can't* smash me! I'm made of some rare metal— plutonium—and I CAN'T BE SMASHED!"

Appalling denouement.

I had discovered what the Alarm Clock symbolized.

It symbolized—myself.

I had been trying to prevent my parents from loving each other.

But that made no sense at all! I had not even known there

was a clock until my throat began to tick—and then I had kept watching the clock so I would not look over at the bed —and anyhow I had not been the clock—I had been that Evil Fur Thing—and I had wet the bed—and I had been an embryo —and anyhow—anyhow——

This jumble of protest slowed down and became bewilderment. What had all these fantasies been about? Why were they all so different, so mixed up, so crazy?

Dr. E obliged by recapitulating the several clock fantasies of the afternoon:

In the first, I had been afraid to look away from the clock over to my parents in bed. When I overcame my fear, I saw that they were asleep—and promptly *got into bed between them.* Then my father woke, was angry, and had mother take me out of their bed.

In the second, when I looked away from the clock over to my parents, I saw that an Evil Fur Thing was *lying between my parents preventing them from making love.*

In the third, I had cried loudly and then wet the bed—because I was not allowed *to be with my parents, in bed with them.*

In the fourth fantasy I again became the Evil Fur Thing *in bed between my parents.* I had tried hard to change back into a baby in the crib but only succeeded in becoming a miniscule creature *lying between my parents,* who then joined both father and mother in their lovemaking. In so doing, I had found tremendous sexual fulfillment—but without the climactic moment. Instead of exploring the reason for that missing moment, I had preferred to return to the clock fantasy, for the fifth time.

And in this last fantasy, the Alarm Clock had tried to come *between my parents to prevent their love:* first by ringing its alarm bell, and when that failed, by becoming a time bomb that exploded mother.

It was then I had cried out that *I* was the Alarm Clock.

At the end of this recapitulation, I was not confused any

more. With dreadful clarity I saw that in each of these fantasies I had tried again and again to come *between my parents and prevent their love.* As a crying baby, as an Evil Fur Thing, as a bed-wetter, as an Alarm Clock, and as a time bomb.

Conscious Me began to protest. I did *not* want to separate my parents or prevent their love. That was absurd. I was a mature woman with children of my own. How could I possibly want to keep my parents for myself, why would I conceivably want to separate them?

The protest stopped because I realized that I and I alone had invented these five clock fantasies.

I could not deny that somewhere within me I was clinging to the infantile wish of keeping both parents for myself.

After this admission, with considerable anger, I demanded to know what GOOD was it to rescuscitate that ridiculous infantile wish? How could it help *anything* to know that as a baby I had wanted to prevent my parents' love?

For answer, Dr. E recommended that I repeat the fantasy still again—but this time, if I were able, to permit my parents to be together and to enjoy their love.

Of course I was able.

For the sixth time I became a baby in the crib, looking away from the Alarm Clock over to my parents in their bed. They were making love. I did not try to prevent them. Instead, once again, I became both my father and mother . . . experiencing their double pleasure which grew stronger and stronger . . . still stronger . . . all-consuming.

Once again I found myself submerging into the sparkling black which was no longer buzzing, nor frightening, but filled with pinpoints of light . . . and I was dissolving into those pinpoints of light . . . yes, I was dissolving out of the matter which was my body into the energy of those pinpoints of light which grew brighter and brighter, obliterating the blackness and becoming a light which was All Energy.

I dissolved into the Nothing which is Everything.

Transcendence.

In the transcendence, revelation:

There was no climactic moment of release. There was no shattering or explosion. There was only further expansion and further fulfillment. It was as if I had become the expanding universe, spreading further and further in every direction, and through the universe of Me there flowed a mighty force, the Life Force, which was like an inexhaustible fountain of fire or air or water, a fountain of eternal replenishment.

". . . That must be why the ancient cities of Europe have so many fountains. To show their people this eternal replenishment."

Unconscious Me had said that and now, one after another, the fountains I had seen in European cities rose before my eyes.

One in particular stood out more vividly than the rest: the tiny Manneken-Pis of Brussels, the little boy who has been flowing without stop for almost five hundred years.

That image too disappeared into the Energy which was sparkling, foam-white, endlessly replenishing, refreshing.

How long did I bathe in that exquisite Energy? Was it hours or minutes or seconds? Time had no dimension in this fountain of fire or water or air.

At length I heard Dr. E say that I might remove my mask, for the session had ended.

I felt that therapy, too, had ended. I had now experienced several kinds of ecstasy. This last seemed far to transcend any physical pleasure I could achieve.

It was as if I had been reborn in that fountain of fire. There was exaltation in me, almost a mystical exaltation. I had not only been freed of my neurosis (a pale and paltry thing now) but I had been permitted a glimpse into beatitude.

I was surprised to hear Dr. E suggest another LSD session.

After these sessions I was never again frightened by a choke-image; not consciously at a dinner party, nor unconsciously in an LSD session, nor semiconsciously as I was about to fall asleep. I was never again kept awake at night by the sound of a clock ticking in my bedroom. I was no longer jarred awake by a constriction in my neck and throat. Finally, the ticking in my throat which had been with me chronically for some ten years disappeared.

Why?

Why was I cured of these several symptoms? How after all is any chronic complaint cured—whether ulcer or phobia or nervous tic or asthma or compulsion—by psychotherapy? This was a question which had puzzled me long before LSD therapy and continued to puzzle me long after I had been pragmatically cured of a chronic tic (the ticking sound in my throat) and a phobia (the sound of a clock ticking in my bedroom *only at night*) and a minor physical complaint (the occasional constriction in my throat as I was about to fall asleep).

Why had I been cured? Eventually I arrived at an answer satisfactory to me.

I believe I contracted those various chronic complaints as the result of one faraway and long forgotten incident:

As a baby, I had seen the act of intercourse which looked to be an act of violence in which father "choked" mother. That scene had so alarmed and sickened me that, as a protection, I had determined "never to feel anything so that I would not be hurt." As another protection, I had determined that, if I were to wake up again during the night I would "keep watching the clock" so that I would not be able to look over to where father was "choking" mother. As a third protection, I "forgot" all about the incident. However, the memory of that incident continued to exist in my unconscious mind which, all unknown to me, evolved further "protections"—in the form of symptoms. I began to tense the muscles in my neck and throat: a protection against being hurt if I were to be "choked." So unconscious was this protection, so unaware was I of this tension, that I never knew it existed until as an adult I took a course in body relaxation and discovered that my neck and throat were being gripped as if in a vise.

There followed a protracted struggle before I could release

the tension. The moment I did, my throat began to "tick": this ticking served perhaps as an unconscious reminder to keep watching the clock so that I would not be able to look over to the bed where father was choking mother. Somewhere along the way, there had evolved a second unconscious protection. I had grown unable to fall asleep with a clock ticking in my bedroom at night. Perhaps the ticking served as an unconscious reminder of the original choking scene. Finally, there developed a third unconscious protection: the constriction in my neck which jarred me awake occasionally as I was about to fall asleep. Perhaps the constriction served as a warning that I might be choked during the night.

With these several unconscious protections, or symptoms, operating in my daily life, I was able to get along fairly well (albeit rather oddly) until LSD therapy when, as the original choking scene came closer to the surface, unaccountable things began to happen. The first was at a dinner party when a guest coming at me as if to "choke" me caused an uprush of unreasonable fear *immediately after which I began to tick loudly.*

As therapy continued and I came closer to the original scene, more and more choke-images appeared to frighten me out of all proportion.

I did not at all understand those choke-images until the last sessions, when I managed to recreate the original trauma. This was not a sudden recall of the event. Rather it was a piecemeal reconstruction, beginning with the moment when the ticking in my throat grew so loud I cried out: "It sounds as if I had swallowed a clock!" In trying to fantasy the clock I had "swallowed," I saw an old-fashioned kitchen clock with a black dial, greenish numerals, and an aluminum alarm bell on its top. I did not recognize that Alarm Clock. But gradually, it located itself near the crib where I had slept as a baby, in my parents' bedroom. I found that I had to keep watching the clock so that I would not look over to where Mommy and Daddy were. After overcoming my fear and looking over at my parents' bed in several fantasies, I came to realize that *what I had seen was not an act of violence but an act of love.*

With that realization there was no longer any reason to be afraid of being "choked," no longer any reason to be disturbed by a clock ticking in my bedroom at night, no longer any reason to constrict the muscles in my neck and throat, no longer any reason for the ticking tic.

And since there was no longer any reason for those symptoms, those protections—they vanished. And I was cured.

That is the answer I evolved, satisfactory to me. But it may not be satisfactory to others. It can very well be argued that this rather complex explanation I have offered is based on one and only one known fact, which was told me by my mother during the course of therapy: that, as a baby, I had slept in a crib in my parents' bedroom.

Suppose mother had never told me that? Obviously, I might never have discovered this early trauma. More than that: It can very well be argued that this early trauma never really happened, and this is an argument I can not refute. I do *not* know if I relived an actual trauma under LSD or if I merely imagined one. Unlike the episode of Miss Leahy whose existence I discovered to be real after I had "imagined" a nurse with a round face, steel-gray hair, and a white nurse's cap trimmed with black, I could never corroborate the existence of an old-fashioned kitchen alarm clock with a black dial and luminous green numerals. I asked both my parents if they had ever owned such a clock but neither of them could remember. I can not then prove the reality of this trauma.

Let us hypothesize that I fabricated this entire infantile episode out of odds and ends of experience. As a child, perhaps I had seen in a friend's home an alarm clock with a black dial and luminous green numerals. And perhaps as a child I had seen a movie in which the villain choked the heroine. And perhaps I had gleaned ominous, violent ideas about sex from books and whispered confidences.

Let us suppose, too, that I began to tense the muscles in my neck and throat after suffering an injury in that area, an injury subsequently forgotten.

And let us also suppose that I was not able to fall asleep with a clock ticking in my bedroom because its rhythmical sound disturbed me, as it apparently disturbs other people. (Many therapists, other than Freudians, report cases of neurotic patients who are disturbed by the ticking of a clock. None of these cases, however, except for the specific symptom, have I found to be similar to mine.)

Finally, let us assume that all of these scattered experiences somehow coalesced in my unconscious mind as a fantasy of a ticking clock in my parents' bedroom which protected me from seeing father "choke" mother.

This would be pure psychic reality and not reality at all. Whether reality or psychic reality, I was cured of several assorted symptoms. That and that alone is the important thing for me.

To test the cure, shortly after this thirteenth session, I deliberately put a loudly ticking clock in my bedroom as I prepared for sleep. As soon as I put out the light, its ticking began to disturb me. But then I reminded myself of the Alarm Clock which I had kept watching so that I would not see father "choke" mother. Then I reminded myself that he had not been choking her. What I had seen was not violence, but love. Gradually the clock's ticking faded into the background and I fell asleep. I have not been bothered by that little phobia since.

I could find no way to test the occasional constriction in my throat, because it did not come back again. The ticking tic in my neck and throat has also gone away. But unlike the constriction, the ticking did not vanish without a trace. Occasionally after these sessions I would begin to tick. When I did, I reminded myself of the ticking clock I had swallowed as a protection against being choked; and I reaffirmed the fact that there had been no choking, no violence; and the ticking would stop. I have not ticked at all in well over two years.

The tension in my neck and throat has proved more obstinate. I am in fact still struggling to break that almost lifelong habit. It has become something of a game with me: when I am involved in some activity—driving a car, reading a book, typing at my desk—I will at times direct my attention to my neck and throat. Invariably a tension is there. Not so complete a tension as when I first discovered it (then it was a stranglehold) but it is a definite tension all the same.

I am still looking forward to the day when I will unexpectedly direct attention to my neck and throat and find that they are *unconsciously* relaxed.

In the week that followed I was far away from the interpretation I have here recorded. Nevertheless, the session I had just had seemed greatly significant to me, for I realized that in many guises I had tried to come between my parents: as a crying baby and an Evil Fur Thing and a time bomb and an Alarm Clock and a bed-wetter. I had clung fiercely to both parents, as if I could not exist apart from them. Until, at the session's end (and at Dr. E's suggestion) I had been able to fantasy my parents as a unit divorced from me, enjoying their privilege of love. In granting them their independence I believed I had achieved my own. That was why I had felt such ecstasy and exaltation; that was why I had felt reborn in a transcendent fountain of All Energy.

Or so I believed.

No recurrence of any symptom came to discredit that belief during the week: no ticking, no need to get up to relieve my bladder before I could fall asleep, no choke-images—not even any insomnia the night before the session. As a result, I went off to Dr. E's office convinced that I had reached the end of the therapy.

16.

The Return of the Full Bladder

THAT conviction grew stronger in the half-hour preceding the fourteenth session; so strong that when Dr. E appeared I announced my cure and proclaimed that I had been psychically reborn.

Dr. E accepted these statements with equanimity.

"Good. Can you fantasy yourself being born?"

Provocative request. Could I?

In a twinkling of the inner eye, I saw myself as a foetus in the womb, drawing nourishment from the umbilical cord . . . and I kept growing . . . a happy vegetable . . . until I was ready to be born . . . but Mother was not going to help me . . . all right . . . I could and I would do it myself.

In fantasy I battered at the narrow opening until it was large enough to push my head through . . . then I slithered and struggled to get my shoulders through . . . after which it was a simple matter to free the rest of my body.

There. I was a newborn baby, slippery with the slime of birth and gasping greedily for air, but I was newborn.

I announced this triumph . . . only to see in the next moment . . . that the healthy newborn baby I was . . . was beginning to shrink . . . smaller and smaller . . . nor could I stop myself from shrinking . . . shrinking into . . . into a four-month-old foetus with a tiny body and an enormous head.

Sickening realization: *in the last session I had crawled inside Mother as an Evil Fur Thing and had become a four-month-old foetus.* Did this mean I was not reborn at all; that I was still an embryo psychically? Conscious Me protested against this symbolism which was much too pat and all untrue. I was not, I was absolutely *not* a four-month-old foetus.

"Then why did you turn back into one?"

Before I could think of a reason . . . I saw the four-month-old foetus returning into the womb . . . reattaching itself to the umbilical cord . . . becoming once more a happy vege-table, absorbing food and life through that wonderful umbilical cord. But gradually . . . some sort of . . . pain? . . . familiar insistent pain . . . what was it? . . . oh no, no . . . but yes, it was. That dreadful full bladder. All over again.

Why? After those many many weeks of frustration, trying to wet the bed in fantasy, I had at long last, last week, succeeded. And since that time I had not once been forced in real life to go off to the bathroom before I could fall asleep. Why should the full bladder have returned to plague me *now?*

No answer but continued distress.

Dr. E suggested that I empty my bladder into the water which surrounded me as a foetus. That seemed a simple solution. But quite definitely and simply I could *not* empty my bladder, not even as a four-month-old foetus.

Same old impasse. And distress. My bladder grew fuller and fuller still. What was causing it to fill up so much? I searched around and found the reason:

The erstwhile wonderful umbilical cord was pouring water into me, a steady and relentless stream of water, through my belly button into my body which was now so swollen that it was going to burst if I could not release the water and I could not release it and I did burst open.

I was a waterlogged dead thing with water pouring out of my nose, my ears, my eyes, out of every hole in my body.

There the fantasy ended.

What the hell had all that been about?

Dr. E recommended that I repeat the fantasy (damn him) to see if I could discover its meaning for myself. I thanked him with sardonic gratitude, stifled my reluctance, and once more became a foetus inside the womb.

Inexorably water began pouring into me from the umbilical cord. Conscious Me recognized this fantasy as a variation of the enema torture: water was being poured into me through the umbilical cord instead of the black enema nozzle, through the belly button instead of the anus, and it had burst me once into a waterlogged dead thing instead of exploding me into a long scream through the tunnel.

But—why? Surely I had resolved that problem . . .

Even as I thought these things consciously, Foetus Me was feeling more and more pain as the water kept pouring into me . . . until the pain became so intense that I could no longer think . . . and there I remained and remained.

Endless time of torture. Finally, abjectly, I asked if I might literally relieve my bursting bladder. I was dumbfounded when Dr. E consented. But I did not stop to question *anything*. I got up very quickly and went off to the ladies' room where I relieved myself completely and effortlessly. Then I returned to Dr. E's office, lay down on the couch, put on the eyeshade——

—and was immediately, overpoweringly assailed all over again by a very painful full bladder.

Horrified, helpless, I begged for one of Dr. E's "clues." He suggested I go with the pain to see if any fantasy would emerge to explain my predicament.

I plunged headlong into the pain . . . and eventually an image did appear . . . dimly . . . was it a statue? . . . of a woman or perhaps a Venus without arms? . . . and without . . . without genitals? I struggled to see more clearly and found that it was definitely a Venus without arms or genitals and where her genitals should be there was only swirling water. . . .

The image faded and I saw nothing more. Probably because the pain was again almost unendurable. Again I begged for a clue, *any* clue, expecting Dr. E to say that I should repeat the fantasy.

He did not. This was one of the rare times he gave me a specific direction. He suggested that in fantasy I give myself a penis.

I recognized this suggestion as Freud's penis envy—a concept which I had always considered absurd and which I still considered absurd.

Tirade: I abhorred such Freudian claptrap; I had never ever consciously or unconsciously wanted a penis nor had I ever wanted consciously or unconsciously to be a boy or man or Lesbian; Dr. E's suggestion was decadent and disgusting etc. etc.

While these condemnations multiplied, I began to remember the times that similar "Freudian claptrap" had proved correct: infantile traumas and sibling rivalry and displacement and psychic reality and puns and . . . and . . . well . . . I supposed I *could* explore this insanity even though I knew, I *knew* I had never wanted a penis. Ever.

This dictum declared, I proceeded with Dr. E's suggestion.

I promptly became a newborn baby boy.

"OK. What am I supposed to do now?"

"Just continue the fantasy."

"But it's idiotic!"

No reply. For some time, I lay outraged. But then the fantasy took over and I saw that I was a baby boy, lying in a crib, playing with his appendage. Next I became a small boy, still playing with it and then urinating through it. No more than that.

I complained that these were routine things to do, and proposed to abandon the fantasy. Dr. E pleasantly recommended that I continue it.

"But what else is there to do?"

No reply.

After a while, I supposed I could be a young man, and promptly became one. He was standing near a bed where a woman was lying, obviously waiting for Him-Me——

At this I rebelled: the entire idea was Dr. E's disgusting and obscene suggestion and I would not continue it, I simply would not. Besides, I *could* not, even if I wanted to which I certainly did not, because I had no idea, none, how it would feel to be a man, physically.

"A clitoris is the vestigial penis in a woman."

Long buried statement from a physiology course suddenly resurrected in my mind. Well, yes, I supposed that clitoral feeling *was* the feeling a man would have—but I was damned if I would indulge that feeling or this fantasy which had been Dr. E's gratuitous and decadent idea anyhow.

Dr. E did not reply.

I cannot remember how it happened (the report is unclear) but somehow or other I did continue the fantasy and became *both* the young man and woman . . . crazy hermaphroditic sensation as the two of us made love . . . sensation which reached a high level of double pleasure . . . pleasure which remained and remained . . .

. . . until the young man was stabbed in the back with a knife.

Who had done that? I turned around and discovered that my father had stabbed me between the shoulder blades and had left the knife there. Extremely painful wound. I struggled to wrench the knife out of my back . . . difficult place to reach . . . but I managed . . . only to have the blood flow more profusely from the wound . . . I tried to stanch the blood but I could not . . . I was going to bleed to death if I could not stop it . . . and I could not.

Suddenly, miraculously, the wound healed of itself. And my back began to develop strong muscles, huge muscles . . . I had the most powerful man's back in the world . . . not only that . . . I had huge male genitalia too . . . what to do with all this maleness?

Sudden simple solution: I would return to the woman lying in bed. Same hermaphroditic pleasure . . . which this time culminated in an ecstatic double orgasm . . . which remained and remained. . . .

Until I was stabbed in the back again, by my father. Again the blood flowed profusely and again I could not stop it. But this time, there was no miraculous cure. The blood continued to flow out of me . . . and the pain grew more intense . . . white-hot overpowering pain which was going to consume me. . . .

From far away I heard Dr. E say: "Remember you're still a man in this fantasy of being consumed."

I wanted to rage at him for his idiotic irrelevance—what in hell did being a man have to do with this white-hot pain?— but I could not speak for the pain. I could only wait until it consumed me, to see what if anything would emerge.

Here ensued one of those seesaw struggles in which the pain occasionally transmuted into pleasure only to revert back into that white-hot pain which never quite consumed me.

Dr. E suggested two ways to break the deadlock: either to use every bit of concentration I could summon to direct the pain, or to relax completely and go with it. I tried both methods, but remained in the limbo of pain/pleasure, which I did not understand at all. Dr. E said it would be better if I could discover what was happening for myself. I agreed but I did not know how to discover *anything*. All I could do was feel white-hot, terrible pain. Implacably vague, Dr. E suggested I create an image of the pain. Gradually . . . I saw it as a white-hot ball of fire in my back . . . which unrolled into a white-hot stream that poured from the wound in my back down through my genitalia . . . an unending stream of white-hot fire or energy . . . which became unendurable.

"I've got to get out of my body, somehow I've got to get out of my body!"

"Why don't you?"

Struggle to break out of the mass of white-hot pain which was my body. Finally . . . finally . . . I saw rising out of the white-hot fire . . . a phoenix . . . I had become a phoenix . . . which then became a vulture . . . I did not want to be a vulture but I was incontrovertibly a vulture, evil and ugly . . .

until somehow . . . the vulture transformed into an eagle soaring through air on great majestic wings. Remarkable sensation for small me to be this magnificent and powerful eagle. Even more remarkable to see the eagle I was flying into the sun where I-He would be cremated and reborn. How would I emerge?

Great expectancy—and disappointment to find, after the cremation, that I had been reborn back into my own body *with that same dreadful pain in the back.*

Angry and bitter protests, countered by Dr. E's suggestion that I disembody out of the pain again.

Once more I managed to dissolve into the white-hot maelstrom . . . out of which emerged . . . the head of a wild woman, one of the Furies. I did not want to be a Fury but there was no help for it, I *was* a Fury flying through the air, blowing up great storms with my mouth. Then the Fury I was transformed into a Winged Victory, a marvelous Winged Victory who had *arms*, and a *head*, absolutely marvelous sensation——

—until I became aware of the pain in my back again. Somehow I had returned to my body and to that damnable white-hot pain which I could not be rid of.

Here I rebelled: I did not understand any of this imagery or disembodiment, symbolically or any other way, and I could not endure the dreadful pain in my back any more. Dr. E asked me to describe the pain. I repeated what I had already said: that it was like a white-hot stream of fire flowing from the knife wound in my back down through my genitalia which were either male or female because I still occasionally felt that crazy hermaphroditic pleasure, but *I did not understand anything and I refused categorically to continue without some explanation.*

"How about trying another fantasy?"

"You mean becoming a man again?" I jeered. "No, thanks."

"Any fantasy you like. Free choice."

I did not mind doing that at all. It would be a delight to

get away from all the self-inflicted torture of the afternoon. What fantasy would I choose?

Before I could decide, I found myself deep in a forest . . . where after a time the young god Mercury appeared . . . lithe and strong and charming, with little wings on his feet . . . and then somehow *I* was the winged Mercury enjoying the beauty of the forest . . . and then a naiad appeared, a lovely naiad . . . and I went to her . . . and we began to make love . . . until an Avenging Angel with a Flaming Sword appeared to confront us. I knew he wanted to stab me in the back but I was not going to let him. I was stronger than he was and fought him off and returned to the naiad——

"But you said you never wanted to be a man, consciously or unconsciously."

Dr. E's remark stunned me. I had been so enchanted with the forest idyll that I had not for one moment realized I had been repeating, in another setting and with other characters, the very fantasy I had repudiated as Dr. E's "decadent and disgusting idea." *I had again become a young man making love to a woman*—and I had so enjoyed the experience that when an Avenging Angel had appeared to stab me in the back with his Flaming Sword, *just as my father had stabbed me in the back with a knife*—I had fought him off so that I could continue making love!

Disconcerting. Very. I refused to accept this denouement. *I did not want to be a man:* I would bring back the Avenging Angel with the Flaming Sword to kill the man I had become. The Avenging Angel appeared. But instead of stabbing me in the back as I fully expected him to do—he castrated me. Literally.

Another disconcertment. Followed by discovery:

In the earlier fantasies my father had stabbed me in the back with a knife, causing a pain which I had described, twice, as a white-hot stream of fire *flowing from my back down through the genitalia.* I had linked by fire the *pain in the back to the genitalia, male* genitalia, for Dr. E had reminded me that I was still a man in those fantasies of being consumed. Obviously, *being stabbed in the back with a knife by my father* was, symbolically, the same as *being castrated by an Avenging Angel with a Flaming Sword.*

These had all been fantasies of castration, then . . . castration . . . what was it . . . Freud . . . castration? . . . but the pain of this newest wound grew so bad that I could not think . . . I could only go with the pain and hope to be consumed again . . . but I was not . . . because the pain gradually transformed into . . .

. . . that old, old full-bladder symptom.

I was right where I had started at the beginning of the session. Or, for that matter, at the beginning of therapy. Right back to the full bladder which I could not release. Painful. Grotesque. Humiliating. And apparently unconquerable.

"What the hell do I do *now??* And DON'T tell me to repeat any more of your goddam fantasies———"

I stopped because the "other voice" interrupted: "I could get rid of that full bladder . . . if I had a penis . . ."

Simultaneously with the "other voice" there appeared in fantasy the fountain of the Manneken-Pis which I had seen so vividly at the end of last week's session; the Manneken-Pis, that little boy of Brussels who has been urinating so contentedly and constantly for almost five hundred years. Now *I* was the Manneken-Pis, and all the unexpelled water that had been plaguing me for the whole afternoon (and for the whole therapy) came sparkling out in a cheerful endless stream . . . dear dear God . . . I really was able to release my bladder now, I really was free of that distress.

And all because I had become the Manneken-Pis with his little appendage. . . .

I found myself giggling uncontrollably at the ludicrous denouement, which proved the Freudian hypothesis I most derided.

Here was the penis-envy theorem. Q. E. D.

I kept on laughing as the water kept pouring out of me in a happy carefree stream.

After my laughter: chagrin. I did not want to be a boy or man consciously. And I was damned if I would be one unconsciously. I would exorcise the man in me. But *how?*

"Why not fantasy releasing your bladder as a woman now?" Dr. E offered a suggestion.

"Oh no!" Involuntarily.

"Why not?"

"I can't. It's impossible." I realized then what the other voice was saying and hastily amended it. "I don't mean it's impossible . . . I mean . . . well . . . I'll try."

I did try. The fantasy was difficult to create at first.

"Well . . . I guess I can . . . but it just seems so dreary . . . it just isn't fun any more."

I began to laugh uncontrollably again. Ludicrous Me, who had always proclaimed my love of womanhood, was now protesting its "dreariness." But I refused to accept that unconscious dictum. And in time, in fantasy, I was able to release my bladder through my own facilities, even with some enjoyment. At which point, Dr. E ended the session.

I left, vastly pleased with the Manneken-Pis revelation and the release it had given me. But I was cautious this time about accepting my "cure." I did not know if the urethral dragon were slain permanently now, or whether he would be resurrected, the way he had been today, in still another guise. I did not know if I had been reborn as a healthy girl baby—or whether I was still a four-month-old foetus of indeterminate sex. I made an appointment for another session to find out.

To anticipate: except for a farewell appearance in the next session, the full-bladder symptom went into the oblivion of the Alarm Clock, the Purple Screw, the Purple Poisonous Peapod and the sundry other symbols of the therapy.

I would like here to give a summation of the full bladder, the most pervasive and persistent of all my symptoms under the drug. It had, in fact, appeared in the very first session when I had begun to feel strong physical desire; only to have that desire transform—astonishingly—into the painful pressure of a full bladder. When Dr. M suggested I "go with" the sensation to see what association would come, I remembered that I had been a chronic bed-wetter as a child. This brought on feelings of shame and disgust beyond which I could not go. (Except to wonder aloud if I were frigid because I was afraid of "wetting" someone, a shameful thing to do.)

In the second session I again began to feel desire which—again involuntarily—transformed into the same full-bladder distress. This time in going with the sensation, I arrived at a totally different association: I remembered the odd compulsion I had developed during marriage of having to get up to relieve my bladder several times each night before I could fall asleep.

In these first two sessions, then, I had evoked two opposite reactions to the full bladder: As a child I had chronically and compulsively wet the bed. As a woman, I had chronically and compulsively *not* wet the bed.

I did not yet know why I had done either of these things. But I did realize, vividly, that in both sessions the pain of a full bladder had cut across and destroyed the sexual pleasure I had been feeling. Clearly my sex problem was linked to this full-bladder problem: but what was the link?

Since I could find no answer by conscious cerebration, I decided to look for an "unconscious" answer in the third session through a fantasy of "wetting the bed." This strategy proved unsuccessful. No matter how I tried to release the full bladder in fantasy I could not: not after five hours of struggle.

Worse: In the fourth session I was not able to wet the bed *either in fantasy or in reality* even though I had deliberately refrained from emptying my bladder for three hours before the five-hour session.

Even though I believed that there was a connecting link between the full bladder and the sexual problem, I could not discover it. Unconscious forces within me were preventing the discovery. Recognizing this fierce resistance, Dr. M recommended other avenues of attack on my neurosis.

By way of those other avenues, in the next several sessions,

I came upon the Purple Screw, the enema, and the Alarm Clock: all of which had been blocks to sexual fulfillment. While exploring these blocks I was never once disturbed by the full bladder—under the drug. But in life it forced me out of bed almost every night. That odd compulsion had returned. And on the eve of the ninth session the compulsion went berserk. Until past six in the morning I got out of bed again and again and again to release the intense pressure of almost non-existent urine.

In the ninth session itself, the first image to come roaring up was an enormous eagle which plucked out my kidney. That eagle plucked out my kidney again and again and again until I recognized in this fantasy the myth of Prometheus and cried:

"Yes, the eagle plucked out his *kidney!*"

I knew very well that the eagle in the myth plucked out Prometheus's *liver,* but I did not realize the mistake until several days later.

Why had I said *kidney* instead of liver? I believe because of *displacement.* I had displaced the *liver* for the *kidney*—which in turn I had displaced for the *penis.*

Preposterous as this may sound at first, I think later events of the session corroborated the hypothesis. For example: The eagle-kidney fantasy brought on *the same full-bladder distress* that had kept me awake the entire night before. That full bladder continued to plague me until Dr. E suggested I displace the bladder pain for vaginal pleasure. Astonishingly, I could. And so completely that for the first time in my life I achieved (in fantasy) a genuine vaginal orgasm.

But—I could not repeat the fantasy. Instead, the full bladder returned, persisted, and translated into a series of dreadful events. My arms began to shriek with pain. Then a buzzsaw appeared to hack off my arms and legs. Then I became the armless and legless Freak crawling on his belly.

(Much later I learned that dreams and fantasies of being deprived of one's arms, legs, teeth, head, or any part of the body are, according to Freud, symbols of castration.)

Finally there appeared a gigantic image of the Purple Screw
—which had been the first symbol of the penis I had seen under
LSD. I proceeded to destroy that Purple Screw—whereupon it
turned into a dish of *kidneys*.

In other words, the Purple Screw, which had originally
symbolized the penis, now became a kidney. Such an equation might read: Purple Screw = penis = kidney. In terms of
this equation, the eagle at the beginning of the session which
had been plucking out a kidney might equally have been
plucking out a Purple Screw or a penis.

This Prometheus fantasy, then, might be considered the
first of the castration fantasies which were to appear.

There were still other kidney episodes in this session which
seem to bear on this hypothesis: I remembered that my sister
had almost died of a *kidney* disease; and that my mother had
had one of her *kidneys* removed; and that I was supposed to
have had a weak *kidney* as a child which accounted for my bed-
wetting. Immediately after these associations I saw in fantasy
that my kidney was badly diseased and that I would have to
replace it if I were to survive. Whereupon the "other voice"
screamed out: "Yes, my father ruined the kidneys of all the
women in his family!" And then I proceeded to remove his
healthy kidney, to give it to myself.

Referring back to the equation Purple Screw = penis =
kidney, I could have been claiming that father had destroyed
all the male organs of the women in his family. (Indeed this is
another Freudian concept: that girl children feel unconsciously
they have been deprived of the organ which their fathers and
brothers have.)

At the end of this ninth session I understood none of these
kidney images. Indeed, I dismissed them as unimportant be-
wilderments surrounding the miracle of the first orgasm I
had ever experienced.

Whatever those kidneys had been meant to symbolize—and
obviously they were related to the full-bladder symptom—I
reasoned since, at the session's end, I had given myself a "healthy

new kidney," the full-bladder symptom would no longer disturb me. And as a matter of fact the full bladder did not appear for several sessions—during which time other problems like the choke-images and the Alarm Clock were resolved so wonderfully that I arrived for the fourteenth session feeling that I had been reborn.

At Dr. E's suggestion I fantasied myself being born as a healthy girl baby—only to regress to a four-month-old foetus which crawled back into the womb to grow again. It was there, as a foetus in the womb, that the full bladder rose up to drown me in water I could not expel. That pressure continued and continued (even after I relieved my bladder *literally*) and might have continued throughout the session had I not begged for help and received Dr. E's "gratuitous" suggestion that I give myself a penis. When at length I brought myself to accept his "decadent and disgusting" idea, I became in fantasy a young man making love to a woman, who was then stabbed in the back. That wound caused a white-hot pain which ultimately transformed into—the full bladder which I could not release.

I still could not conquer that damnable and devastating full-bladder symptom.

Out of this dismaying realization, came the information from my "other voice" that I *could* release my bladder *if I had a penis*. Whereupon I became the Manneken-Pis, releasing all the unexpelled water of the whole afternoon, and the whole therapy, in a carefree sparkling stream. From that moment (except for a last appearance in the next session) I was permanently rid of the full bladder.

In the beginning of therapy I had discovered that there was a connecting link between my sexual problem and the full bladder, but I had not been able to discover it. Now, in this fourteenth session, I had. The link was a strong unconscious protest at not having a penis with which I could let go and release the fluids inside me, as the Manneken-Pis could do.

Penis-envy theorem. Q.E.D.

I would like to anticipate a valid objection: that this unconscious penis envy did not come to me spontaneously—it came only *after* Dr. E put the idea in my head.

That is true. It was only because Dr. E gave me the specific suggestion that I became in fantasy a boy baby, a boy, a young man, the god Mercury, and ultimately the Manneken-Pis.

Suppose Dr. E had *not* given me the suggestion? Several other solutions are possible: I might have suffered many more sessions of full-bladder torment before I arrived at the penis-envy denouement. Or I might have suffered the full bladder indefinitely without ever arriving at a resolution. Or I might have arrived at a totally different solution had I been left to my own devices.

It is very possible that I arrived at a *wrong* solution of the full-bladder symptom because of Dr. E's suggestion. But again, whether reality or psychic reality—it does not matter. The fact remains: I was cured. Just as I was cured of the ticking in my throat whether because of an imagined Alarm Clock or a real one, so was I cured of the full bladder.

In the interests of truth, I was not completely cured of the symptom. At rare times, when I am overtired, the full bladder returns and I give in to it rather than struggle against a disagreeable pressure which would only tire me more.

Even so, I am grateful to Dr. E for his "gratuitous suggestion" which when he offered it seemed preposterous. And I confess: this unconscious-penis-envy solution still seems preposterous to me at times—when I have only my rational mind with which to draw conclusions, and not the remarkable double awareness which is granted under LSD.

In routing the full bladder, all unwittingly, I opened a new —and final—battleground of unconscious conflicts. But I did not know that, and lived a rich, unproblemed life during the interval—until the night before the session.

Twice that night I was frightened awake by two nightmares, two different nightmares, neither of which I understood. I remembered both when I woke in the morning, however, and determined to explore them in the session.

17.

The Bitten-Off Nipple

SHORTLY after the half-hour began before the fifteenth session, I decided to explore the first nightmare, to interpret it myself, if I could:

In this dream, a primitive, powerful country had invaded the United States and I had found refuge, together with friends and relatives, in an underground shelter so well provisioned and camouflaged that we could survive the duration of the war there comfortably. Unexpectedly, enemy shock troops attacked the shelter. My friends and relatives scattered but I was captured and forced aboveground, where I was ordered to round up those who had escaped. As soon as I did, I realized, these barbarian shock troops would destroy us all——

At which point I had wakened from the nightmare, in terror.

Now, about fifteen minutes after having taken the drug, this dream which had been incomprehensible spontaneously revealed its meaning:

The *underground shelter* was obviously meant to be a symbol for my unconscious mind which existed below the surface and had been *so well camouflaged* that it could survive indefinitely without being discovered.

My friends and relatives in the shelter were symbols too—of my symptoms and neuroses which could have *survived the duration comfortably* had not those barbarian shock troops discovered the underground hiding place.

Those *barbarian shock troops*, I quickly realized, were symbols again—and very apt symbols—for Doctors E and M who were using the *barbarian* (experimental) *shock* therapy of LSD. They had already forced my unconscious aboveground, and were now asking me to *round up those friends and relatives* (symptoms and neuroses) that had escaped. As soon as I did round them up, we were to be destroyed.

As this interpretation unfolded, the nightmare lost its terror and became instead an encouragement: unconsciously I might be frightened at losing my neuroses but consciously I was delighted.

This discovery could not have taken more than a few minutes, because there was still time remaining of the first half-hour. In that time I decided to explore the second nightmare, which was far different and proved to be far more difficult:

In it, an unknown and loathsome dark woman came to visit me, after having discovered that I had been having an affair with her husband. In retaliation, she demanded that I have a homosexual liaison with her——

At which point I had again wakened, this time feeling horror and disgust, as well as bewilderment for this inexplicable dream.

Now, under the drug, it was *still* inexplicable. I had never had any kind of homosexual dream before, nor had I ever had any kind of homosexual experience in life. Why, then, this dream? (Oddly and obtusely, I did not connect this dream of homosexuality to the previous session when I had again and again fantasied myself *to be a man*.) As I tried to penetrate its meaning, the same disgust and horror I had felt on waking from it returned and intensified—which was when Dr. E joined me.

I told Dr. E the first nightmare and my interpretation, with which he seemed to agree. When I began to tell the second, I found myself stuttering, and then became mute. I recognized these two old resistances and refused to succumb to them and eventually succeeded in telling the whole of the dream. Whereupon I immediately (and *effortlessly!*) voiced the usual protests: the dream was absurd, I had never had any homosexual desires, there was no possible way to understand or interpret this dream, it was lunatic and meaningless, etc., etc.

Dr. E proposed that I try to understand its meaningless absurdity by re-experiencing it now as a fantasy.

Outrage at his suggestion—which I promptly swallowed because the suggestion was so clearly sensible: what better way to interpret a dream than by "dreaming" it under LSD?

Again and again I tried to recreate the nightmare. But each time I conjured up an image of the loathsome dark woman, she either disappeared into the buzzing black or changed into Heaulmière or became some acquaintance whose problems I began to discuss. All these transformations, I realized, were forms of resistance which I fought off, one by one, until I was able to maintain a clear image of the repulsive Dark Lady (emphatically *not* of the sonnets) who then insisted that I get into bed with her.

Again, horror and disgust.

But eventually I was able to do as she asked. When I did, most oddly her body grew enormous while mine grew smaller and smaller, almost microscopic. Then Microscopic Me began crawling up the mountain of her body, higher and higher, until I reached the top—which proved to be the nipple of her breast.

Whereupon I became a baby. Literally a baby.

I could hear gurgling sounds come out of Real Me as in fantasy Baby Me began to suckle at the breast . . . but the more I suckled, the hungrier I became . . . ravenous . . . I simply could not get enough milk . . . frustration growing more and more intolerable . . . until out of the frustration I began to bite down with my toothless gums . . . biting down harder and harder . . . and as I did . . . I grew afraid, very afraid . . . and unaccountably afraid.

Now Real Me was making whimpering sounds which, as my fear increased, turned into a baby's loud wailing.

From very far away I could hear Dr. E ask what was frightening me, but I could not answer him because I did not have any words with which to answer and besides I did not have any idea *at all* of what was frightening me. I looked around and around to find the reason but I could find nothing.

Unexpectedly, in the high tones of a baby, my other voice complained that there was no more milk and that my brother could have all the milk he wanted but when it was my turn Mother had no more milk and it was not fair and if I was a boy I could have all the milk I wanted just like my brother——— .

And with that—the full bladder returned.

Horror at its return.

(I could not know, of course, that this was to be the full bladder's farewell appearance. Nor did I appreciate until recently that it returned *at just the moment I was complaining that I was not a boy like my brother*. Full bladder = penis envy. Again Q. E. D.)

Horror of the full bladder compounded with jealousy of my brother compounded with anger at my mother because she did not have enough milk. These emotions coalesced around my toothless mouth . . . which developed small sharp teeth . . . which began to bite down hard . . . harder and harder still . . . until in fantasy . . . I bit off the nipple. Blood gushed over me from the mutilated breast. . . .

I was sickened by the wicked thing I had done. I was a monstrous baby. Evil. This self-loathing focused now in the full bladder which grew infuriatingly painful—*and which I could not release.*

"Why can't you?"

"I don't know, damn you!!"

A stream of invective against **Dr. E** and his hapless therapy that did not cure anything. When the invective subsided to a trickle, Dr. E asked again what the block was.

Suddenly—I saw it.

It was the Bitten-off Nipple, blocking my sphincters.

In fantasy I pulled it away, and then all the fluid inside me began to flow out in a fine free stream. Release. Relief.

Followed by total bewilderment. Why had that dreadful full bladder returned? And why, of all the unlikely symbols, had it been blocked by a Bitten-off Nipple? I could make nothing of anything.

Dr. E volunteered one of his rare explanations: As infants, he told me, we sometimes feel hate and rage against our parents, who seem like omnipotent gods. (I recognized this analogy immediately: in my fantasy, the Dark Lady had grown gigantic while I had grown so tiny that I had to crawl up her mountainous breast to reach the nipple.) However: as infants we do not dare express our hate and rage for fear of being punished. Instead we repress these destructive and "evil" impulses—and we also feel *guilty* for having had them.

I found this explanation reasonable but wildly *un*satisfactory. All right: some thirty years after the fact I had gotten around to expressing infantile hate and rage—but what the devil did my hate and rage have to do with the dream of homosexuality I had been trying to interpret?

Dr. E suggested I find out by repeating the fantasy.

With much unwillingness I returned to the Dark Lady. Whereupon I became a baby again. And then the baby became a four-month-old foetus who crawled back into the womb and attached itself to the umbilical cord to grow again. Swiftly the foetus reached full term and wanted to be born. But the Dark Lady would not help the birth. All right. I decided to manage things for myself and I did. When I emerged, I found that there was no one there to help cut the umbilical cord.

Undismayed, I cut the cord myself and then tied it. There. I was a healthy newborn baby girl.

Conscious Me watched anxiously for fear the baby girl would turn back into the four-month-old foetus. . . . She did not: she *remained* a healthy newborn baby.

I announced this fact in triumph to Dr. E—who answered that I had neatly evaded the problem of homosexuality which I had set out to explore. I protested and pointed out, with some perspicuity, I *still* believe, that I had carried through both fantasies and had found the "homosexuality" to be an aspect of the mother-child relationship. The first fantasy had explored the problem of feeding, which was connected to jealousy of my brother. And the second had explored the problem of achieving independence of the mother.

Dr. E did not seem convinced for he asked me to repeat the fantasy. I obliged him and returned to the Dark Lady. This time, surprisingly, her husband appeared—and proved to be Dr. M. Forthwith I decided to have a liaison with *him* and fantasied an experience of sex-and-love which culminated in ecstasy.

How many times now, in how many fantasies, had this wondrous thing happened to me? Ecstasy which lingered and lingered, without reaching a climax. Enviable state, certainly. But I grew dissatisfied: what was blocking the climactic moment?

"What do you think it is?"

"I don't know."

"I do."

"Oh, you're so damn smart!" Again I was furious with Dr. E. "You sit up there on that chair with its bird's-eye view. Pretty easy from up there to see what goes on!"

"Why not try it?"

"I will!"

In fantasy I switched places with Dr. E and reviewed the events of the session leading up to this moment of unreleased orgasm. Clear as clear could be, I saw the block. It was the same Bitten-off Nipple. Before it had blocked the sphincters. Now it was somewhere deep in the core of me, blocking the flow of orgasm.

In fantasy I pulled it away and—from deep deep within me a great fire of feeling burst through, consuming me. I exploded into a thousand thousand shimmering particles.

An infinity later, those myriad particles reassembled back into the entity of me, which was exceeding puzzled:

"But—I don't understand . . . ? What was that Bitten-off Nipple doing *there?*"

Naturally Dr. E wanted me to answer that question for myself. I studied the Bitten-off Nipple, certainly one of the oddest of symbols, and tentatively ventured that it might represent my guilt and evil because as a baby I had wanted to mutilate mother . . . ? Yes. The Bitten-off Nipple represented the Evil in me, which had been a block to sexual fulfillment.

So: Guilt for the Evil in me had proved to be still another block to fulfillment. How many blocks had I found so far? However many, surely there could be no more. Not now. I had had too many complete, glorious experiences under the drug. . . . I lay back, bathed in the glow of liberation: I was whole, well, and a woman.

For once Dr. E seemed to agree. At least he proposed a totally new fantasy: I was to imagine a house of several rooms, each of which contained a specific threat to sexual fulfillment. I was charmed with the suggestion, for it seemed a kind of graduation exercise; one which I was confident of meeting. I believed I could face any threat—and overcome it.

I tried the fantasy, but could not create an image of a house with rooms. Instead I slipped down into the buzzing black— which no longer frightened me—and waited calmly to see what threat would appear.

It was the Cedar Chest.

I remembered how afraid I had been as a child that the Freaks would come out of the Cedar Chest and attack me. I also remembered the nightmare of my very fat aunt, freaklike because she had only the upper half of her body. That nightmare, I then remembered, had been a displacement of my unconscious wish to hack at Mother's stomach and destroy the baby she was carrying.

The Cedar Chest, then, represented my *guilt* for such a murderous impulse, and my *fear* of retribution. I had been afraid that the Freaks would come out of the Cedar Chest to attack me, *just as I had wished to attack Mother.*

But I no longer had that wish, consciously or unconsciously. I no longer felt guilty and I was no longer frightened by this image of the Cedar Chest. No. I had exposed the threat and disposed of it.

As if on cue, the Cedar Chest faded into the buzzing black——

—and was replaced by the armless and legless Freak crawling on his belly with a knife between his teeth. I recognized this Freak from the horror movie I had seen as a child. I also recognized him to be—myself.

How many times in how many fantasies under the drug had I seen myself similarly deformed? On several occasions, a buzz saw had *hacked off my arms and then my legs.* I had been a Venus without arms with only swirling water where her genitals should be. I had been a baby in a basket, with the head of an adult. . . .

Gasp, as I suddenly remembered that in this very session I had become a baby *crawling on its stomach* in just the way this Freak was now *crawling on its belly.* Startling parallel: in the movie, the Freak had been crawling to attack and mutilate the villainess; in today's fantasy, as a baby, I had been crawling to attack and mutilate Mother's breast. . . .

Both fantasies, apparently, represented the same wish: to mutilate and destroy the Omnipotent Evil One.

But I no longer had that wish consciously or unconsciously. I was free of this threat too.

Obligingly, the armless and legless Freak evaporated into the buzzing black.

Two down. Which would pop up next?

A door appeared in the blackness. I opened it in fantasy, and as I did, in reality, my arms flung themselves across my chest as if they had been pinned into a strait jacket.

Oh, but I knew this threat well. This was Miss Leahy pinning my arms down so that I would not scratch at the measles and/or chicken pox. But I had misinterpreted her act as a punishment for "playing with myself." And so dreadful had that punishment been that I had utterly repressed all memory of "playing with myself," of masturbation, until the age of eighteen or nineteen.

But I was no longer afraid of being punished for sex. As if to prove I was free of the fear, my arms unfolded themselves involuntarily from across my chest and began to wave about freely. This was a sensation I enjoyed enormously—until the very freedom of my arms reminded me of the terrible tensions they had suffered, tensions which had evoked the two inexplicable sentences: "I feel as if I were about to burst or explode" and "I'm a long scream through the tunnel." Those tensions and those sentences had been symbols of a second childhood trauma: the too strong, too hot enema.

As if in corroboration, the slim black Enema Nozzle appeared in the sparkling blackness. And I remembered how that Enema Nozzle had transformed into a red-hot poker, an acetylene blowtorch, a Flaming Sword, the Purple Screw and the Purplish Poisonous Peapod. All of these had been expressions of the one terror: that I would be tortured and then exploded into "a long scream through a tunnel" if I were to be penetrated by an Enema Nozzle, or indeed by any other foreign object.

Now I knew, unconsciously and consciously, that being penetrated need not be painful. Quite the contrary. Now I knew the wondrous pleasure of being penetrated in the act of love. I was free of this threat too. Completely free.

Exhilaration now. And confident anticipation. What next?

Again a door in the blackness, and again I opened it——

And immediately felt a sharp pain in the back.

Oh yes. That pain in the back represented the recent fantasy in which I had become a man, only to have father stab me in the back with a knife. Symbolic castration. But I had disposed of this threat too. I no longer wanted to be a man. I was free of that unconscionable desire.

But even though I had announced my freedom, disconcertingly *the pain in the back did not go away.* In fact, it grew stronger. So strong I felt it would destroy me if I did not stop it. And I could not. I was helpless against the pain.

Why?

No answer. Only pain.

Eventually Dr. E suggested that perhaps I had not yet worked through my desire to be a man. I scoffed through the pain: of course I had, I was delighted to be a woman, absolutely delighted!

"Then why doesn't the pain in your back go away?"

Infuriating question because I had no answer to it. More infuriating when the pain grew so intense that I could not speak at all.

Then, in a blur of pain, the Avenging Angel appeared with his Flaming Sword. Good. He would castrate me again, and that would delight me, because I hated being the man I had inexplicably become now in the fantasy.

Stupefaction in Conscious Me, as the man I had become in fantasy categorically refused to let the Avenging Angel perform the operation. Why did He-I refuse? The "other voice" answered that He-I were not in the least sorry or guilty to be a man; in fact we were proud of the privilege.

Conscious Me would brook none of that nonsense, deliberately called back the Avenging Angel, and this time submitted to the Flaming Sword.

Whereupon white-hot pain spread through me like fire . . . it *was* fire . . . and I was being consumed in the fire . . . like a torch . . . I was a flaming human torch . . . like one of those early Christian martyrs who had been burned at the stake. . . .

Good God. Was this torture-and-martyrdom what I unconsciously equated with surrendering my "manhood"? Apparently it was, because this fantasy had sprung from me, *me* and no one else.

I hated this Christian martyr image I had created, *but I could not change it*. I remained and remained a human torch. . . .

How to conquer this insane wish to be a man?

Charging up from the depths a new, vivid fantasy: I was pinned down on an altar. Sacrifice in a Black Mass. Hundreds of black-robed, black-hooded priests in attendance. Standing over me, the High Priest who was also covered with black hood and robes, but whom I recognized to be—Dr. M, holding a razor in his hand, with which he was going to—castrate me.

Oh good God, not again. . . .

Dr. E interrupted to ask what a Black Mass meant to me. I

answered impatiently, "All that is evil," and went on with the fantasy. I did not realize until weeks later that I had equated being castrated—deprived of my "manhood"—with "all that is evil."

I began to struggle, to break free of the bonds that tied me to the altar, but the High Priest summoned another priest to pin me fast, and again I was powerless to move. (It is fascinating that the imagery of being *pinned down* appeared here again. It would seem that the original trauma of having my arms *pinned down* when I was a two-year-old baby, so that I could not move them, imprinted itself so strongly on me that I repeated the experience in many variations and contexts throughout the therapy.)

Incongruously this second priest was dressed in casual sports clothing, the only one of the hundreds who was not dressed in the black robes and hood. I looked up at his face and discovered him to be—Dr. E. I giggled: apparently my unconscious did not believe that Dr. E was as sadistic as other men.

This sidelight amusement was abruptly extinguished when in fantasy Dr. M began the operation, an extremely painful one, particularly when he continued with the razor to cut into me, to turn me into a woman. Even then the ritual was not complete, for I was now to be possessed in turn by each of the hundreds of priests. I cried out that sex should never exist without love but Dr. M ignored me and performed his part of the ritual with absolute impassivity. Then it was Dr. E's turn. Unexpectedly, with Dr. E, I began to feel pleasure. Not the wondrous pleasure I had known under LSD but the unsatisfying clitoral pleasure I had often experienced in life. Unsatisfying—and deliberately created, I realized now, by *contracting* down there. Why was I contracting? Why had I done that in life? I did not know.

In the next moment I discovered why: for by contracting still tighter I saw in fantasy that I had cut off Dr. E's member which was now inside me.

Pungent realization: I had castrated Dr. E by those contractions which I had recognized from my sexual experiences in life. Were those contractions I had so often made an unconscious desire to *castrate?* This disturbing thought led to an even more disturbing one: After so many fantasies of *being* castrated, I had now in this fantasy *been the one to castrate.* I had reversed roles: instead of being the masochist, I had become the sadist. But I did not want to be either, for both roles were dreadful——

Dr. E interrupted to suggest I stop intellectualizing and continue the fantasy instead.

Relieved at not having to pursue this newfound Evil, I returned to the Black Mass—only to find that the hundreds of priests had disappeared. I was alone now, but still feeling that unsatisfying clitoral excitement——

Because, I realized, I was still contracting tightly. I deliberately released the tension.

And when I did . . . my womb began to open out . . . the way a flower does when it blossoms . . . yes . . . in fantasy now my womb was a flower . . . a gardenia . . . like one of the ones in bloom outside my home . . . and nestling in the heart of the gardenia . . . most bizarrely . . . was Dr. E's cut-off member . . . which now changed into . . . a buzzing bee . . . not an ominous but a friendly buzzing bee who fertilized the gardenia.

Miracle of conception: miracle of a tight green bud appearing in the heart of a stem-leaf, bud unfolding into the whitish-green, then ivory of a radiant gardenia.

Dr. E asked what had happened to the bee.

I looked and saw that the bee was flying off because there were so many other flowers that needed to be fertilized.

"And I'm perfectly happy to let you go off to your other patients," I heard myself say. I understood then, and only then, that the bee had been Dr. E. And for once, Conscious Me and Unconscious Me were in agreement: we were content for Dr. E to leave, now that we had unfolded into the blossom of womanhood.

III

My Self and I

18.

The Scared Spermatozoon

With the fifteenth session, I had faced the various threats to fulfillment which I had discovered under LSD—and had overcome them. Even the most recalcitrant of these threats, my unconscious desire to be a man, had apparently been resolved with the blossoming gardenia, symbol of my acceptance of womanhood.

As a matter of fact, in reality, I began to feel transcendentally well. Daily experiences would take on an unexpected radiance. One day, for example, driving through a street in the neighborhood, I was captivated by the red-orange mass of a flowering eucalyptus tree. That tree had been on that street all the years I had been driving through it, but I had never seen it in blossom before. Probably because I had never really looked at it. Now I did. And I saw that it was beautiful. Another day I was so entranced with the aquamarine color of a swimming pool that I seemed to become one with the aquamarine; the feeling was almost like religious communion.

Children on their way to school, a bluejay in the backyard, salespeople and supermarkets—I looked at these commonplaces, and found them transformed.

They had not changed. I had. Everything, I discovered all over again, everything is in the eye of the beholder.

But I did not trust my new-found beatitude. I did not know

whether I had been "twice-born," to use the religious terminology of William James, or, to use the current terminology,
whether I was in a temporary "manic" phase which would
swing back into a customary depression.

To find out, I asked for another session—and was chagrined
to learn that I had not at all conquered the pain in the back,
symbol of my unconscious desire to be a man.

In retrospect it is obvious that I had accepted the gardenia of
womanhood only after the most dire tortures: after being a
ritual sacrifice at a Black Mass, a Christian martyr burning at
the stake, a young god castrated by an Avenging Angel with a
Flaming Sword.

None of these could quite be called a joyous acceptance of
womanhood. But I did not realize this fact until the next session. And it required several strenuous sessions before I was
able to resolve the battle of my two sexes.

In the course of that battle, I was forced to wrestle with the
Evil in me, which gave rise to self-loathing, which in turn made
me seek out a sadistic love who would punish and reject me.

I had long been aware of my penchant for falling in love with
someone who did not return my love; a penchant I deplored
but could not control. In these last sessions I learned to control
it, and I learned to accept myself as a woman, and to overcome
my self-loathing, my bisexuality, and my need to be punished
by an Unrequited Love.

These later explorations may seem incredible, for they led me
into a stranger, perhaps deeper level of the unconscious. Rich
and extraordinary imagery appeared to me—but it was imagery
which did not seem related to my specific life history. It was
as if I had gone beyond Freud's *personal* unconscious into the
collective unconscious of Jung—a realm of which I had only
the vaguest knowledge at the time.

This was not an abrupt transition. Actually, in the last few
sessions already described, I had stepped across the border. For
example, the repulsive Dark Lady was no one I had known personally, nor did she ever evolve into someone I had known but

forgotten, like the nurse with round face and steel-gray hair who proved to be a very real Miss Leahy. No. The repulsive Dark Lady remained and remains an Abstract Woman who, in her darkness and repulsiveness, might very well be the Jungian *archetype* of the Evil within one's self. Another, similar archetype might be the Evil Fur Thing which had already appeared, and was to appear again and again.

These had been rare occurrences in a fantasy life which had been based primarily on *personal* experiences. Now such images were to appear much more frequently. In facing these phenomena, I was able at last to achieve a fusion between my self, and me. This fusion was, I believe, the specific factor which made my cure as permanent as it has proved to be.

Much of the material of these last sessions is irrelevant to therapy and is omitted, so the reports of the individual sessions are considerably condensed. Also, since I felt consistently well during this period, I have not described the intervals between sessions.

I arrived for the sixteenth session with no specific area to explore (except the general question of whether or not I had completed therapy); nor had I had any dreams during the week to furnish a clue. As a result, in the first half-hour, I let my fancy roam free—and continued to do so with Dr. E, when he appeared. This freedom evoked remarkable imagery, irrelevant to therapy, for a considerable time.

But then, gradually, I began to feel afraid. This fear, which I could neither define nor understand, grew so strong that I tried to embody it in a fantasy.

Almost immediately there appeared in my mind's eye—the sculpture of the Laocoön, great snake coiled around a father and his two sons who are struggling to break free.

What did the Laocoön mean in relation to my fear?

Dr. E suggested I might find out if I were to keep watching it. I did . . . and somehow became one of the sons struggling to get free of the snake . . . but the snake was too powerful . . .

implacably it wound itself around my arms and then my body until I was powerless to move. Again my arms had been pinned down, and I was paralyzed!

Then the snake stared at me with one bright-yellow malevolent eye, while I lay helpless, waiting to be crushed to death. But the snake did not crush me.

"What is the snake doing?" Dr. E asked.

"Oh, not *again*——!"

My "other voice" had wailed those words at just the moment, in fantasy, that the snake began to nibble at me down there where—I had become a man again. Of course: I had been one of the *sons* in the Laocoön. And now I was being castrated by the snake. Then the snake continued to nibble into me, to turn me into a woman. Again.

Sudden illumination: This Laocoön fantasy was like the Black Mass fantasy of the session before, in which the High Priest had castrated me, and then turned me into a woman. Now it was the snake that performed those operations. But why?

Even as I asked, I knew: because I still must have that unconscious desire to be a man.

"But I don't! I mean, I got over that nonsense the last time when I became a gardenia. I mean—I DON'T WANT TO BE A MAN, I REALLY DON'T!!"

"Then why did you have this Laocoön fantasy?"

"Oh, damn you!" Dr. E's question was infuriating—because unanswerable. "Why can't I just be a woman and be *happy* to be a woman? I am, consciously. Why can't I be, *un*consciously?"

Even as I complained, the Laocoön snake in fantasy began to transform into . . . the Evil Fur Thing . . . which grew monstrously large . . . and became a succubus . . . its innumerable brown tentacles reaching out to . . . to *me* . . . ingesting me into itself . . . completely ingesting me.

Whereupon . . . *I* became the Evil Fur Thing, sinewing through the sparkling black, infinitely disgusting and infinitely evil. There the fantasy ended.

But what had it meant? Again I knew, even as I asked. I had

been the Evil Fur Thing, because of my corrupt and incorrigible desire to be a man. How to overcome that desire?

Strong appeals for Dr. E's help elicited one of his "hints": that I fantasy someone All Woman.

This suggestion disconcerted me, for just a few nights ago at a party I had been asked whom I considered All Man and had had no difficulty with an answer. But when I had been asked who was All Woman—I could think of no one.

I tried now, under the drug, to think of someone who was all that is feminine. I considered women historical like du Barry and Cleopatra; women mythological like Juno, Diana; women half mythological like some of the current movie stars—but none of them seemed a satisfactory embodiment of womanhood.

Discouraging realization: I had no concept of femininity, either consciously or unconsciously.

Dr. E suggested I fantasy an Abstract Woman who would be everything feminine.

After several unsuccessful attempts, there evolved in my mind's eye a naked full-breasted woman, lolling on her back. She was of Rubensesque proportions, and seemed All Woman—but she was two dimensional, a black and white lithograph. I wanted her to become flesh and blood.

Long struggle before this Rubens woman came alive. When she did—she wanted love.

Obligingly an Abstract Man appeared——

And the Abstract Man was—ME.

I did not want to be a man, I did not! Why did my unconscious insist on turning me into one?

Dr. E suggested I continue the fantasy. I did, and became BOTH the Abstract Man and the Abstract Woman: weird and wonderful to be these two Rubensesque creatures who grew to godlike proportions as they consummated their love. Double ecstasy—out of which there issued a spray of white foam, thousands of sparkling drops of foam.

I became one of those drops, which proved to be a spermatozoon. The Spermatozoon that I was began racing toward an ovum, racing faster and faster—until suddenly he veered away, his tail frantically wiggling.

"He's awfully frightened."

"What's he afraid of?"

I did not know, and asked the Spermatozoon why he was afraid. I seemed to hear him say that if he were to go into the ovum he would lose his tail and die.

(I did not appreciate until later that this was still another fantasy of castration. The Scared Sperm was afraid *he would lose his tail*—which is exactly what had been happening to me in these last sessions.)

I answered that of course he would die, and so would the ovum, but in such death lay transfiguration; for then a new life would be created, and there lay the miracle of evolution. My argument apparently convinced the Spermatozoon, for he reversed course, raced back toward the ovum—and penetrated it.

Miracle of a fertilized ovum; splitting into two, four, eight——

But Dr. E, damn him, stopped the fantasy—for he now wanted me to become an ovum about to be penetrated. I agreed, became an ovum—and immediately grew terrified when I saw the Spermatozoon racing toward me, for I realized that if he entered me, I would be destroyed.

Again Conscious Me offered the same argument: that in such death lay transfiguration. Again the argument proved successful, for when the Spermatozoon came charging toward me this time, I welcomed him . . .

And exploded into millions upon millions of electric sparks. In the very nucleus of those millions of sparks—a crystal-like drop of fire which seemed to contain the secret of creation. If only I could penetrate into it, become one with it——

But the fire-drop faded. Nor could I recapture it. I was left bereft, but exalted. And then puzzled. What had been the meaning of that exquisite fantasy?

Dr. E wanted me to interpret it for myself.

I found it necessary to review the events of the session, beginning with the moment I had felt an undefinable fear which I had fantasied as the Laocoön. Watching the Laocoön, I had become one of the sons whom the snake had pinned down, castrated, then turned into a woman. This fantasy, I had realized, had been a repetition of the Black Mass fantasy. Both had demonstrated that I still unconsciously wanted to be a man.

In trying to overcome that incorrigible drive, I had created an Abstract Woman who represented everything feminine. This Abstract Woman had wanted love, and promptly an Abstract Man had appeared—and proved to be ME. Further repetition of that unconscionable desire to be a man.

In the act of love, however, I had become BOTH the Man and the Woman. Did that mean I was at least *bisexual* now?

"What came out of the union?" Dr. E asked.

"Oh. . . ." Weary realization.

A spermatozoon had come out of the union. And a spermatozoon, obviously, could never be anything but male. So I had gone around still another circle, and arrived back at that damnable, unconscious desire to be a man.

With this realization the pain in the back appeared. With the pain, sharp futility: I would never overcome this desire to be a man. Never.

"I'm stumped." My other voice had spoken those words. Conscious Me, hearing them, burst into laughter. All unwittingly, I had made another pun: for, in these last sessions I had been repeatedly castrated, I had quite literally been *stumped*.

Hilarity superseded by confoundment. How the devil could I get rid of Masculine Me?

I would have to wait for another session to search for an answer.

19.

The Malevolent Maggot

THE night before the seventeenth session I was shocked awake by a nightmare in which I had been engaging in homosexual practices with the repulsive Dark Lady. Shock, revulsion. Followed by the realization that this nightmare had been still another expression of my unconscious desire to be a man.

(Obtusely, I did not connect this nightmare with the one of two weeks ago, in which the repulsive Dark Lady had made her first appearance, demanding that I have a homosexual liaison with her. I had not obeyed her request then, but had waked in horror. In this nightmare, which would seem to be a continuation of that first one, I had been carrying out her order.)

I could not at all understand why my unconscious masculine drive should have expressed itself in a nightmare of *homosexuality*. I determined to explore the reasons in the session.

With the typical perversity of my conscious mind, I forgot all about the nightmare until half the session had gone by. When I did remember it, the usual diversionary tactics: stuttering, mutism, buzzing black. I fought these off, reported the dream, and then gagged with disgust.

Why that nightmare? It would be impossible to feel anything remotely like love for the repulsive Dark Lady. Such an act was the antithesis of love. It was pure self-abasement. Why had I dreamed that dream??

For answer, a vague image of an insect, perhaps an ant. Then, in fantasy, my father appeared, saw the insect, and stepped on it. I heard my other voice say that I deserved to be stepped on and killed because I was so vile.

This unconscious comment startled me into the realization that *I* had been the insect. As if in corroboration, the insect reappeared in my mind's eye. This time no one came to kill it. Instead it grew larger, more loathsome. I saw now that it was a maggot. And the maggot was—ME.

The Maggot that I was approached my father, attached itself to his body, drained his blood, and ingested him into itself. Then repeated this dreadful process with my mother. Then with my brother. Then with my sister.

All of my family had now been devoured by the Maggot. And now it squatted in the blackness, bulging red with all the blood it had consumed. I hated the Maggot and longed to destroy it, but I did not know how. After a time, the Maggot transformed into a vulture equally malevolent who tore and ate the raw dead flesh of people and looked around for more bodies on which to feed. Abruptly, the vulture changed into a creature that might have stepped out of an Hieronymus Bosch painting: stork legs, bird body, face of human flesh which wrinkled and sagged into a great craw of a mouth. It walked around so proudly. It was so disgusting. Eventually this creature, too, transformed into——

—the Evil Fur Thing which maneuvered its infinitely long brown body with its innumerable tentacles through a void of blackness to . . . ? I did not know where it was going, but followed the Evil Fur Thing until it arrived at its home, which proved to be the caverns of Hades. Here the Evil Fur Thing sinewed its way through limitless labyrinths where black rivers flowed. On the banks of the rivers grew black gardenias with white leaves. These were the Flowers of Evil, beautiful in their perverse way.

I found—with considerable shock—that I was enjoying myself as the Evil Fur Thing in these labyrinths of Hades.

Why? Why was I enjoying myself? Why, indeed, had I seen myself not only as the Evil Fur Thing, but as the vulture, the Bosch monster, the Malevolent Maggot?

These images led me directly back to the repulsive Dark Lady and to the original question: Why had I dreamed that I was involved in infamous union with her, a union which represented all that was Evil?

The Dark Lady was obviously the equivalent of these monsters—but, equally obviously, so was I.

Why? I had no answer.

20.

The Gorgon

WHY was I those creatures of Evil, equivalent somehow to the repulsive Dark Lady—and to Masculine Me?

For answer, obligingly, the Malevolent Maggot appeared,
squatting in the blackness, bulging red with blood. Gradually,
superimposed over the Maggot, there appeared an image of my
brother as a small boy, and then myself, as myself. I saw that I
approached my brother, hacked at his body, and stuffed it into
the Cedar Chest. I proceeded to do the same with my sister.
There, I heard myself say, *now I can be both a boy and a girl*
and my parents will love me alone. Instead, in fantasy, my
parents appeared—and were furious. (I could not in the least
blame them.) They pinioned my arms and legs against a wall,
and threw sharp, pointed darts at me. End of fantasy.

Which I could interpret without any help:

I had been the Malevolent Maggot because, as a child, I had
apparently wanted to kill off my brother and sister, so that I
could be *both a boy and a girl,* and have my parents to myself.

This explained my unconscious desire to be a man: I had
wanted to replace my brother.

It also explained why I had been the Creatures of Evil: as a
child, I had wanted to murder my brother and sister. (And,
being so evil, I had to be punished. In this fantasy, I had even
conjured up my most usual form of punishment: first, I had

been *deprived of my arms and legs,* and then I had been *penetrated by sharp and painful objects.*) Clear as clear could be.

But: I no longer wanted to be rid of my brother or sister. I no longer wanted to be both sexes. I did not feel evil, and I did not want to be punished. Why this fantasy at all? Had I not, several sessions ago, been reborn as a healthy *girl* baby, and remained a healthy girl baby without regressing back to a four-month-old foetus of indeterminate sex?

As I made this protest, I saw in fantasy, again, that healthy girl baby. And she began to change . . . but not back into a four-month-old foetus. No. This time her wrinkled newborn face transformed slowly into the wrinkled face of an old old man with a large nose and gold-rimmed glasses . . . familiar face? . . . dear Lord . . . it was the face of . . . Mahatma Gandhi. What in the name of all that is holy was Mahatma Gandhi doing in my fantasy? (This image of Gandhi, I later learned, might be described in Jungian terms as an archetype of the Wise Old Man.)

Before I could find out, the Maggot returned—and ingested the baby-who-was-Gandhi into itself. I hated the Maggot for doing that, but the fait was accompli. And because it was, I realized, a transformation was now going to take place in Maggot-Me. . . . Gradually the top of the Maggot's body was lifted up . . . as if it were being pushed open from inside . . . which it was . . . for out of the Maggot's body . . . there emerged a lovely young woman, made of marble. Slowly her marble body became flesh and blood. And now she was clad in a Greek chiton, and she was carrying a dagger and shield. She was some sort of warrior. Yes. She was an Amazon. I knew she was an Amazon because one of her breasts had been removed so that she could better carry her shield.

(This was an odd fact I had somehow remembered from a lecture heard long ago: the word "Amazon" is derived from the Greek words *a mazos* meaning "without a breast." I reported this esoterica to Dr. E and added with a chuckle: "Well, I guess I'm making some progress. At least I'm permitting myself to be a woman now, even though I'm allowing myself only one breast.")

The Amazon seemed to be going on a mission, which I seemed to sense was to cut off the Gorgon's head. Fearful mission, for the Gorgon was supposed to transfix into stone whoever looked upon its face. Yet the Amazon was unafraid. She sought out the Gorgon, who was concealed deep inside a cave, and she looked upon its face—and she was not turned into stone. Instead, the Gorgon was the one to be frightened, for it retreated. But the Amazon pursued it, caught it, and expertly hacked off its head with its hair of living snakes—all of which promptly died. Then the Amazon picked up the head and carried it outside the cave to take it to . . . where? I did not know, but followed the Amazon until she arrived at . . . Dr. E's office.

The Amazon (who was now myself) threw the Gorgon's head at Dr. E's feet. He nodded, and stepped on the Gorgon's head just as my father had stepped on the ant in the previous session. Then Dr. E dismissed me, saying that he must go on to his other patients. End of fantasy.

Well. . . . Had it been so easy to get rid of Evil Me? Was I really to be discharged from therapy? For answer, Dr. E asked what the Gorgon's head symbolized. I had to admit I had no idea. Dr. E offered another of his "clues": that I look into the eyes of the Gorgon.

Fire-yellow eyes, blazing with hate and rage and jealousy . . . and those fire-yellow eyes were . . . MINE.

Crazily, I had become the Gorgon, full of rage and hate. I heard myself say that I wanted to destroy Dr. M because he always punished and rejected me.

(Here I interrupted the fantasy, delighted at my unconscious perspicuity. Of course I had to "destroy" Dr. M, symbol of the Unrequited Loves in my life: of course I had to be rid of that masochism. At this juncture, it seems, I was going beyond the problem of bisexuality into the problem of my need for a cruel, punishing "love.")

Returning to the fantasy, I saw that Dr. M was falling into a sea of blood . . . where he was going to drown . . .

But before he could drown . . . I saw myself diving into the sea of blood to rescue Dr. M . . . to bring him to a sandy white beach . . . there to give him artificial respiration.

Whereupon I stopped the fantasy, realizing that I was trying now to *revive* the Unrequited Love. Stupid. Once and for all, I must rid myself of that masochism.

So I returned to the fantasy—and found, with relief, that I had not been able to revive Dr. M after all. He was quite quite dead. I stood up on the sandy white beach. Alone. And free.

I walked along the beach, enjoying my freedom . . . and came upon a dark forest . . . and entered the forest . . . and found that it was beautiful, carpeted with a multitude of violets.

(Here I interrupted the fantasy again to remark that the violets were the same color that had threatened me in earlier sessions. But now, with considerable vainglory, I announced that this violet color was no longer threatening, but inviting.) Having made this remarkably *in*correct observation, I returned to the fantasy where I proceeded to lie among the violets, to wallow in their fragrance and sensuousness.

After a time, I wanted someone with whom to share their beauty.

Inevitably—Dr. M appeared.

It is difficult to believe, but in this trice of time I had *completely forgotten* that I wanted to be rid of Dr. M once and for all. What is even more incredible: I was delighted at seeing Dr. M, and delighted in our love.

Ecstasy of interpenetrating with him and with the violets and with the forest; then the ecstasy of dissolving into a field of pure Energy, the Energy which exists before it becomes Matter. Here—a series of extraordinary images, unrelated to the specific problem.

Only at the session's end did I realize that I had not at all destroyed the Unrequited Love that punished and rejected me. If anything, by interpenetrating with Dr. M, I had intensified that drive. Stupid, destructive thing to do. For if I did not rid myself of this masochism I would probably find someone new to punish and reject me, just as Dr. M, and William, and Arthur had done.

How to be rid of the dreadful pattern?

21.

The God of Wrath

AGAIN, the night before the nineteenth session, I was frightened into wakefulness by a nightmare which consisted of just one sentence: "C—— R——'s son is the thing that terrifies me."

Eerie sentence, and incomprehensible, for I knew C—— R—— to be an unequivocal Lesbian who never had had a son. Yet: "C—— R——'s son is the thing that terrifies me."

(I realize now that this nightmare was the last of a trilogy. The first introduced the repulsive Dark Lady who demanded homosexual relations (which were prevented because I woke up). The second showed a consummation of that union. And this one, the third, revealed the product of the union. (But this insight came only much later.)

But what did that mean?

In the session I tried again and again to fantasy who or what C—— R——'s son might be. No success. Instead a profusion of imagery unrelated to the problem.

Toward the end of the session (*again*, and in spite of my conscious determination *not* to pursue an Unrequited Love) I somehow became involved in ecstatic union with Dr. M—out of which union I conceived. When the child was born, he emerged full blown as a great bull of a man, bellowing with rage and brandishing a club in his hand. Spontaneously I christened him the God of Wrath (and not for a moment did I recognize that he might well have been C—— R——'s son).

The God of Wrath began to suckle at my breast, but he was such a bull of a man, this newborn son of mine, that he sucked first my breast and then all of me into himself—whereupon *I* became the God of Wrath, and *I* began to bellow with hate and rage and jealousy.

Bewilderment. Why had *I* become the God of Wrath? I did not know until Dr. E asked what I, as the God of Wrath, wanted to do.

"I want to kill all the men who have rejected me!"

My other voice had spoken those words. And now in fantasy as the God of Wrath, I embarked on an orgy of murders, killing Arthur, William, Dr. M, my brother, my father. . . .

When I had done with the orgy, when I had spent all my rage and hate and jealousy—futility.

I had murdered these men again and again in earlier sessions, only to have them return more alive and alluring than ever. Only last week as the Gorgon, I had drowned Dr. M in a sea of blood. But a little later *in the very same fantasy*, he had reappeared, and I had succumbed to him all over again.

(This fantasy of the God of Wrath was identical, thematically, with the previous week's fantasy of the Gorgon whose "fire-yellow eyes had blazed with hate and rage and jealousy" before he had destroyed Dr. M. The only difference in these two fantasies was that the God of Wrath was more ambitious than the Gorgon. He destroyed *all* of the Unrequited Loves in my life, not just Dr. M. But again, this insight came only in retrospect.)

How could I *genuinely* destroy my need to be punished and rejected by Dr. M, or William, or Arthur?

Dr. E suggested that the solution lay, not with those men, but with the earliest of my Unrequited Loves: with Father.

I answered with considerable bad temper that I had learned that particular Freudian lesson thoroughly in psychoanalysis.

What I had not learned, and apparently would *never* learn, was how to apply the lesson.

No. I was incurable.

This pronunciamento made, I asked for another session. Another chance to cure the "incurable."

22.

Empty Ecstasy

SINCE I had no idea how to attack this problem of the Unrequited Love, and since I had had no fantasies or dreams during the week to give me a clue, I decided to begin the session by following Dr. E's suggestion: I would go back to my first love, Father, to discover if I could what had started me looking for punishment and rejection.

Deliberately I created a fantasy of myself as a little girl at home with Father. But as the fantasy developed I found that I wanted to leave home, and Father, to look for a new love which would be free of punishment and rejection.

I set out on an unfamiliar road which led after a time to a plateau, carpeted with fine fine sand, red and delicate under a piercing blue sky.

(Here I remarked that this plateau was *not* an imaginary but a very real plateau I had stumbled upon during a recent vacation. And I congratulated my unconscious for having chosen such an exquisite place to know a new and healthy love. Again I had made, unknowingly, a remarkably incorrect observation: I had chosen as a setting for a new and ideal love—a plateau of *red* sand and piercing *blue* sky. *Red* and *blue* combine, of course, to make the violet color which had so consistently threatened me—and which continued to threaten me, as this fantasy proves.)

I sat down on the fine red sand to wait for an "Ideal Love": a man who would neither punish nor reject me but a man who would return my love.

Dr. M appeared.

Again it is difficult to give this credence, but I was delighted by his appearance and insisted that this was Dr. M "without his sadism." So strong was my capacity for self-delusion; so strong was my unconscious need to seek out rejection and punishment.

As Dr. M approached me, however, he somehow transformed into Arthur, the first man with whom I had "fallen in love" only to be rejected. Now Arthur became enormously attractive, just as he had been years ago when I first knew him. I had to struggle against his attractiveness now, just as I had done then, when our relationship had proved too destructive. Eventually I managed to get free of him and to send him off the plateau.

"There," I heard myself say. "Now I can go back to Dr. M without his sadism."

I turned back to Dr. M—only to find William. I was forced to struggle against William now, a struggle even stronger than the one with Arthur—and a struggle which proved unsuccessful. For when William claimed that I still wanted him, I could not deny it. Worse: when he offered me sex without love, I accepted his offer and entered into a union with him which culminated in orgasm: endless, ecstatic—and empty.

Nothing, nothing emerged from this union. The emptiness of never-ending ecstasy.

At length, evolving out of the ecstasy, a memory: Years ago I had read of a scientific experiment in which electrodes had been placed in the brains of mice. The sensation evoked was so pleasureful that the mice had remained and remained in that state, even refusing to eat—until eventually they had starved to death.

Insight: In this fantasy I had been doing exactly the same thing that the mice had done. I had been remaining and remaining in ecstasy with William—*even though I had been determined to be rid of masochistic, unrequited love.*

Only after this insight was I able to break away from William, and send him off the plateau.

There. Now I was free. Free to find a good and healthy love.

Sudden bewilderment. I had no idea where to find such a love. Beyond that: I could not believe that a man existed who was capable of a good and healthy love.

Dr. E reminded me that this was a fantasy and that I could *invent* such a man. Yes. I could and would invent one. Only after considerable perseverance was I able to create this Abstract Man—who turned into

Dr. E.

During the lengthy interval of creating this Abstract Man, Dr. E, somehow the pain in my back had returned. This was a most unexpected development for I was not in this fantasy striving to be a man, nor had I been castrated. Why had the pain come back? For answer, most oddly, the Dr. E I had created in fantasy (NOT the Dr. E who was sitting near me) explained that it was not necessary to suffer the pain any more; nor was it necessary to find an ideal love to be rid of the pain. All I need do was to channel the pain, a destructive force, into a constructive force which I could pour into my writing, or relationship with my children, or into social activities. . . .

As this Dr. E of fantasy spoke, he began to look more and more like a friend of mine, an actor whom I had seen recently in two performances. Gasp of discovery. In both performances, my friend had played the role of—*a priest*.

New insight: I had equated a "good and healthy love" with the love of a *priest*—which of course could never be sexual. Apparently, unconsciously, I could not conceive of an ideal love which included sex. With this realization, the pain in the back grew worse.

And the session ended, with the problem still unsolved.

23.

The Grand Canyon

THIS was perhaps the most sterile of all sessions.

In the beginning, I recreated that exquisite plateau of red sand and blue sky, hoping to find an Abstract Man with whom I could share an ideal, *and sexual,* love.

For an interminable time I could invent no man at all.

When at long last I was able to fantasy such an Abstract Man, he became—inevitably——

Dr. M.

And—incredibly—I united with him. And I found ecstasy. Again.

But this time the ecstasy (as it had been with William) was *empty.* Until, piercing through it, the pain in the back.

Again, bewilderment: why the pain again?

For answer, I seemed to see my body as the continent of America and the pain in the back as the Grand Canyon. I tried to penetrate into the depths of the Grand Canyon, to find the source of the pain.

But it was bottomless, fathomless, impenetrable—just like the pain in the back.

This was as far as I could go in the session. Which was no-where at all.

24.

The Riddle of the Sphinx

THE pain in the back came back again and again
during the week as a very real and painful physical complaint.
Baffling, not to say annoying, phenomenon.

At the beginning of this session, I complained to Dr. E of this
new development. He offered a tentative explanation: That the
pain had appeared in recent sessions after I had felt "empty
ecstasy" with one or another Unrequited Love. Perhaps, Dr. E
continued, the pain which had originally symbolized the punishment of being deprived of my "manhood" now symbolized
another punishment—being rejected by someone who gave me
sex without love.

This explanation struck me as cogent. But *unhelpful*.

*What could I do to be rid of the pain, to be rid of this un-
conscious drive to be punished?*

Dr. E recommended that I transform the pain, a destructive
force, into a constructive one. I retorted that his proposal was
more properly a riddle for the Sphinx than for me, a woman
of limited intelligence. Whereupon I settled down to try to
solve the Sphinx's riddle.

Immediately and appropriately, the pain in my back appeared, surely a destructive force. In fantasy, I tried to turn
it into a constructive force, and saw it promptly as an electric
blowtorch with which I was trying to burn my way through a

very thick wall of steel. Eventually I did burn a tunnel through the wall, walked through the tunnel, and emerged—into blackness. In the blackness, slowly, a fire appeared. I walked into the fire and found in it a flight of fiery steps. I climbed the steps and found at the top a large and fiery keyhole. I walked through the keyhole and emerged—into a clear blue sky. In the sky, an enormous, beautiful butterfly perched in ecstasy. As I watched, the wings of the butterfly dropped off, and out of its body emerged——

—the heroine of a movie I had recently seen, a heroine who deserted her nice young fiancé for a sophisticated man who after a time treated her cruelly and rejected her.

Chuckles of weariness and futility. I had gone round and round and round, lo these many circles and had come back each time to the same old stand. I was still fantasying punishment and rejection from the Omnipotent Sadist.

Dr. E recommended that I try the fantasy a second time. I did, and found a procession of superb images, irrelevant to the problem.

Only at the session's end did the pain return—violently— to remind me of the problem for which I had been unable to find an answer.

25.

My Self and I

I HAD now devoted seven full sessions to this inter-woven problem of my unconscious desire to be a man, which had elicited images of myself as creatures of Evil, which Evil I kept striving to punish by seeking out (all unconsciously) an Unrequited Love who would punish and reject me.

Four sessions ago I had felt that I was incurable. Now I was sure of it, and said so to Dr. E at the start of the session. He answered pleasantly that he did not think I was incurable. I countered, unpleasantly, by asking what facts warranted his inane optimism?

Dr. E began to explain by pointing out that I had been fantasying not only masochistic tortures (being burst open, drilled with blowtorches, castrated) but also sadistic tortures (I had been the one to burst open, to castrate)——

I interrupted, annoyed at his inane observation. I *knew* I was both masochistic and sadistic. But I did *not* know how to over-come either disgusting drive. Did *he?*

For answer Dr. E suggested that I create a fantasy of myself as a child which would embody *both* drives.

I probably would have scoffed at this "inane" idea too—had there not appeared, with astonishing swiftness, an image of my father as a man of white-hot fire, beating Mother with a cat-o'-

nine-tails whip, beating her until she dissolved into the air. Then Father transformed gradually into a Sphinx with the paws of a lion: around the head of the Sphinx appeared a halo of light, which I recognized as a symbol of Mother. . . .

Fantasy stopped.

I remarked, with contempt, that I had invented a fancy little fantasy of sado-masochism—which had taught me nothing.

Dr. E observed that I had not put *myself* in the fantasy: what would happen if I were to watch Father beating Mother?

Most unexpectedly I began to cry, to protest that I did not want to put myself in the fantasy, I would not, I just would not—but then I *was* in the fantasy, watching Father as he beat Mother . . . and then . . . to my wonderment . . . I saw myself step between Father and Mother . . . to hold back Father's arm so that he could no longer wield the whip. Even though he was far stronger than I was, even though he could destroy me . . . I was not afraid. Somehow I knew I could stop him . . . not by physical strength . . . but by . . . it seemed by . . . staring into his eyes? . . . yes, staring into his eyes, compelling him to stop, compelling him to turn away. . . .

As he turned away in fantasy, I felt a surge of power, unsuspected power: *I had challenged evil in someone stronger than myself, and I had won.*

Thrill of accomplishment. This solution was a far far better one than the childish device I had been using, of *murdering* the Omnipotent Sadist (the Unrequited Love). Pride of accomplishment.

Until Dr. E asked how I could apply this new-found principle, practically, in life situations: either with the Unrequited Love, or with other forces which I might judge to be evil.

A spontaneous new fantasy erupted in my mind:

Michelangelo's superb sculpture of David . . . whose marble body now changed into the flesh-and-blood body of a lithe young man, armed with slingshot, ready to battle Goliath . . . and somehow . . .

I became David.

In the fantasy, most confusingly, I was not only David now, but I was also myself, a woman—suffering the pain in the back. Swiftly, the pain transformed into a lion, which lion I recognized to be my father, or Dr. M, or any Omnipotent against whom I had always felt powerless. Again, I felt powerless against the lion. I *was* powerless, it seemed, for the lion began to devour me—until David appeared, to rescue the woman from the jaws of the lion. When David set the woman down, she turned into a Brueghel peasant, coarse and unattractive. David did not like her, and left her for new adventures. But before he could go far, the lion reappeared and attacked another woman whom I again recognized to be myself. Again David rescued the Woman Me. This time when he set her down, she became a fat old hag with greedy eyes, whom I spontaneously christened Avarice. David disliked Avarice, and harangued her until she promised to share her wealth. Then he left her for new adventures.

But Dr. E suggested that David now rescue myself, *as myself*, from the lion. Suggestion adopted. As David, I rescued myself from the lion. But as David, I did not like myself and prepared to leave. In one of his rare directives, Dr. E asked me *not* to separate David and the woman. In fact: he asked me to unite them.

Ridiculous request: which of the two did Dr. E want me to be in this romance? David-Me or the Woman-Me? It seems he did not care. Chortles at the absurdity, insanity of this romance with myself. But, with high humor (since no fantasy is impossible under LSD), I agreed to contrive this love affair, just to please Dr. E.

For quite some time I could *not* contrive it. David kept turning back into a marble statue. Impossible to have a romance with a marble statue. Then, when he remained flesh and blood, he refused to have anything to do with me. Since this was *my* fantasy, I did not accept this dictum, and eventually created a David who loved and wanted me just as I did him.

Somehow . . . somehow . . . in the act of love . . . I became both David the Man and Myself the Woman. Together we reached ecstasy, twin ecstasy. And together we dissolved, in ecstasy, into the Energy which exists before Matter. And there, in pure Energy, was All-Knowledge, miraculous realm where I wanted to linger and linger——

But Dr. E would not permit me to linger in abstract All-Knowledge. He wanted me to absorb a specific piece of knowledge: to find out what had been causing the pain in my back.

Gradually, it became clear what had been causing the pain (which had appropriately returned when Dr. E mentioned it):

In every human being, I seemed to be told, there is a fire that burns, a creative fire. When that fire is permitted to burn freely, the human being is healthy and creative, whether he be farmer, artist, mother, workman. But when the fire is blocked, as it is by this pain, then the person is crippled, just as I had been crippled for most of my life. As a child, I had felt worthless because I did not have my brother's masculinity and intelligence, nor my sister's grace and beauty. And because I had felt worthless I had withdrawn into non-identity and non-feeling.

Later in life I had found one worthiness: a talent for acting. But I had used the talent as a means of escaping into the identity of the characters I portrayed, instead of searching to find my own identity.

Later, when I turned to writing, I had in some measure abandoned non-identity. In writing, I had tried to probe into who and what I was, hoping in the process that I could find out who and what other people were, for we have in each of us, all of us.

Unfortunately these last few years I had been dodging that search, and compromising for hack work and money. But I would not do that any more. I should, and would, work creatively. I should, and would, write about this extraordinary experience of self-discovery under LSD.

"I can stand straight now, and let the fire burn freely inside me."

As I heard myself speak those words, the pain in my back disappeared. And I knew that it had gone, permanently.

For in this last fantasy of David and the Woman, I had united the two conflicting parts of my being. No longer would one part of me punish and reject the other. I had combined the two separate heritages of my father and mother. I had fused the masculine part of me with the feminine.

In other words: at long last, My Self and I had become one.

Epilogue

Now

Now

PEOPLE who have known about the therapy have eyed me curiously—for I do not look any different—and have asked if the treatment helped me. What they have really wanted to know, though not in these words, is whether my self and I have lived happily ever after?

The answer is, of course, no.

A great scientist once said that each new answer to a problem merely paves the way for further, more difficult questions. He was referring to the realm of physics, but the same principle seems to apply to people. If, for example, we succeed in answering our basic needs for food and drink and shelter, then we are faced with other, more difficult needs—for security, or status, or love, or fame, or self-expression. Ever higher and higher levels of problems struggle to find solution, spiraling further and further out into the vastness of that which has not yet been accomplished.

On a very small scale, so it is with me. My old needs have been met and satisfied; but now I find that there are new needs to be met which, if satisfied, will in all probability give rise to further needs as yet unknown. It is somehow right that this should be. "Ah, but a man's reach should exceed his grasp, or what's a heaven for?"

Before therapy I was always grasping—and futile grasping it

was—for the man who would fill the void within me. This was the pivotal point around which my life revolved. Now that pivotal point has shifted. I no longer feel a desperate emptiness inside. Instead I feel capable of coping with my problems, in my own way. I do not mean, of course, that I no longer want the companionship and love of a man. I do, very much. But I no longer want a man to protect and punish me; I no longer want a man just like the man who married dear old mom. I want someone with whom I can share life's experiences, however difficult they may prove to be.

This change of focus has wrought a transformation in the way I live my life. I do not now meander through parties and people in search of the other half of me. All the psychic energy I had been spending so extravagantly is now available for two quite different pursuits.

One of these pursuits is in the area of my work. Previously, as I have explained, I was a writer of slick fiction. I was aware that this was a trivial occupation but it was one which furnished a livelihood for my children and me.

Toward the end of therapy I grew to realize that I did not have to earn so much money in so frivolous a way. I wanted instead to write this book. But I knew that writing such a book would be a gamble with the odds enormously against me. What publisher would accept it? And even if a publisher were found, who would read such fantastica? Had I myself read this sort of book three years ago I would have hooted derision at "that same old Freudian stuff."

Nonetheless I determined to write the book because I believed my experience to be an excellent example of how unconscious processes affect one's daily behavior and emotional life. Having made the decision, I realized how ill equipped I was to write the book. My ignorance sent me back to college, to take course after course in psychology, physiology, learning theory, and theories of personality. The more I studied, the more fascinated I became with this frontier of scientific exploration: the interrelation of body and mind. So fascinated that I continued studying, received a degree in psychology, and am currently enrolled as a graduate student in the hope of eventually doing research along this frontier.

And here am I, a middle-aged woman back in college. I feel a little absurd, and more than a little bemused. It is not an easy pursuit. Not too long ago I listened to a professor outlining a course in physics, in which he mentioned the "transposing and factoring of formulae," "the exponential function," and how "ten to the minus eighth was a reciprocal term." The eighteen- and nineteen-year-old students around me were nodding their heads in perfunctory agreement, but I was agape, as if listening to a foreign language. Perhaps my dilemma is more cogently described by this recent incident. My son, now in his first year of high school, brought me his algebra paper to correct, for by this time I had completed a course in college algebra. I could appreciate that he had arrived at the right answers, but I did not understand the process he had used and said so. He was puzzled as he exclaimed: "But Mom—that's the multiplicative identity!" I could only look at him with awe as he went on to tell me about that day's lesson in general science, which had dealt with the uncertainty principle as it is applied in atomic physics, and Millikan's oil-drop experiment, both of which he explained to me with far more clarity than I could have explained to him. Apparently the knowledge I am acquiring with so much difficulty at college is already being taught, more fully and comprehensibly, to children in the ninth grade.

Clearly there has been a knowledge explosion in the years I have been away from school, and I do not honestly know whether I shall be able to cope with the work. This is one of the problems I am facing as I pursue my new goal. But here is the golden fact: I can accept these new problems without panic and with whatever resourcefulness is within me. Indeed, I face each day as a glowing challenge. Will I be able to master probability theory? Will I be able to integrate the contributions of Miller or Mowrer or Murphy into a better understanding of human nature? I think about these things as I drive to school each morning. And sometimes, even as I drive and ponder, I find myself all at once overwhelmed by the color of a beech tree, or the formation of clouds against a hill, just as I did when I was seeing the world through the mists of LSD.

That is one great area of change in my life. There is another. No longer are my children on the periphery of my awareness. I am now able to give to them the love I had been squandering on the Omnipotent Man. It is a far more beneficent use of love. And not only is more love available to them, but more understanding. For instance: like most children, my daughter has a great longing to fly. Not long ago she told me of a "funny dream" she had had, in which a bird had flown into her bedroom and promised to teach her how to fly. All she had to do, it seemed, was to put two fingers into the two holes where the bird's wings were. She did, and unexpectedly there were scissors in those holes which cut off her fingers.

Three years ago I would have smiled and said, "Yes, that is a funny dream," and promptly dismissed it. Now, after my experiences with the Buzz Saw and the Black Mass and all those other fantasies of castration, I can still smile and say, "Yes, that is a funny dream"—but I believe I know what the dream is meant to symbolize, and I am not at all alarmed. For I know my daughter's unconscious fantasy of castration, according to Freud, is normal for her age and development. Furthermore, with luck and a fairly decent life, she need never know that those unconscious fantasies existed, much less what they may have meant. Bernard Shaw once challenged Freud, saying that he had never to his knowledge been in love with his mother. Freud's reply was that there was no reason why Shaw should ever have been aware that he was, a remark which caused Shaw to look relieved and comment: "Oh, so that's what you're getting at."

My son has had an interesting dream, too. Actually it is a recurrent nightmare in which he finds himself at school when the Third World War begins. The alert sounds, and he is told to lie flat on the ground. The bomb starts to fall, and he awakes

terrified. Now that he has begun puberty, the dream has recurred but with this change: He is in school, the war starts, the
alert sounds, he lies flat on the ground—and the bomb does
fall. He is killed and ascends into the sky where God judges
him, and judges him to be good, so that he is allowed to be
born again.

This new development in the dream seems a hopeful and
healthy one. I believe that my son is unconsciously facing the
crisis of changing from boy into man, and that he is able to
"be born again" into manhood. Perhaps I am only indulging in
amateur psychoanalysis. I cannot say.

But I can say that I enjoy my children, and enjoy spending
time with them. This summer the three of us went on a long
planned month's holiday abroad. I was aware that traveling
abroad with two children could be difficult, and at times it was.
We laughed and cried our way through a blizzard in the Alps
in August, the paucity of taxis on a bitterly cold night two miles
from our hotel, a sudden attack of "turistica" in the ladies'
room of a theater, and no hotel accommodations on arriving in
a totally strange city after having traveled, awake, all through
the night. I am pleased that I was able to meet each emergency
as it arose. More than that: we all had a wonderful time.

To recapitulate: before the LSD experience, I was a writer
of foolish fiction, going through rounds of casual parties and
people, having an unsatisfactory liaison with a man who did not
want me, and more or less ignoring my children.

Today I am a graduate student of psychology, without a man
but without the frantic need for one, enjoying hugely my roles
of mother and middle-aged college girl. I hope eventually to
have a career in scientific research, although whether that goal
can be achieved remains to be seen. Meanwhile, my life has
new savor, new meaning—and new mystery.

Appendices

APPENDIX A:

LSD-25

THIS is a first-hand report of an LSD experience:

Tchaikovsky's Violin Concerto was playing, and suddenly the music became unbelievably beautiful. I, who am known to have two tone-deaf ears, could feel the music to such an extent that it became one of the most beautiful experiences of my life: it was complete fulfilment. . . .

I closed my eyes and saw patterns of indescribable colors which kept flowing one into another. These exquisite patterns whirled and circled inside me in rhythm to the music. When the record finished I became almost violent in my demands for more music. The time between changing records, which could have been only fifteen or twenty seconds, felt like an hour. During that brief time I opened my eyes and looked at a painting on the wall. It showed a firing squad of four rebels shooting two people. As I watched, the six people in the painting came to life. Sometimes they fought with each other and sometimes they danced with each other. Then the music started again and the exquisite patterns began once more. Now I felt detached from the visions. Almost as if I were not a person, but rather as if I were part of the beauty of the universe. Of creation . . .

I began to think about atomic theory, and the sameness of the microcosm and the macrocosm. It was as if I saw the structure of the universe, and I saw that the positive and negative charges within an atom are the only building blocks, out of which grows everything that exists.

Suddenly my mind raced through from the beginning to the end. I went through evolution, from the original explosion through primordial worlds in which I felt myself to be a reptile, a bird, a beast; on until the first independent thought was created in the mind of the beast. I stood up and walked to a mirror. I saw in myself the face of an ape—and also the master of the world. . . .

A new wave passed over me, and I felt that in a second I had lived through a lifetime. Time seemed to be completely collapsible, and a strong feeling passed through me that everything that had ever happened or will ever happen was happening at this moment. . . .

Next morning, all the effects of the drug were gone, with the exception of my appreciation of music. I believe that the drug helped to remove a block in my mind. Almost everybody in my family was extremely musical, and I had been forced to take piano lessons at a very early age, which I hated. Possibly this rebellion had made me "tone-deaf"—and possibly LSD ended the rebellion.

In conclusion: The experiences I had under LSD I consider to be among the most profound of my life.[1]

This is the LSD experience of another person:

. . . Dr. R had changed: his head was more than twice its normal size, while his pelvis had shrivelled up horribly. He began shaking his pelvis at me in an obviously sexual way. To my left, Dr. W was clearly smirking behind his hand to the nurse. . . . I was hopelessly trapped. . . . The very walls were closing in on me, and even the furniture was part of the plot. A chair suddenly tipped over so that one leg pointed at my heart. . . .

I turned away from everything and smashed my fists into the pillow. Then I launched into a long and varied stream of obscenities. . . .

"Dr. W is here," the nurse said suddenly out of nowhere, and it occurred to me that this was the answer. . . . As it turned out, though, Dr. W only wanted to ask questions.

"Do you feel faint? People around you seem funny? Strange taste in your mouth? Hot? Cold? Color? Shapes?"

. . . Of course, that's the way they do it, you know: they pretend to be kind and understanding to break you down. Then they cut you up into pieces with questions. Note for future reference. Watch out for questions. . . .

With Dr. R it was no better . . .

"Now tell me the meaning of this statement . . . People in glass houses shouldn't throw stones."

I had heard that of course a thousand times, yet just now the meaning eluded me like a shifting silvery snake.

"Watch out for broken glass," I finally managed to say, but somehow that didn't seem quite right. . . .

It was now eminently clear that Dr. R intended to jeer at me . . . I turned my head . . . and spat right at him. . . . A mistake. For now, Dr. R, his face a terrible mask of hatred . . . holds boldly in his hand a small strange sort of dagger, silver and blue as it catches the light. Now their heads are suspended over the bed like ugly giant balloons or huge rotten cabbages. . . . Now . . . pain, pain, pain . . .

I began to gain sanity and control, undoubtedly [because of] the hypodermic of Thorazine which had been administered. As a doctor, I am glad I got a glimpse of the echoing terror that is insanity. But as a man, I know I will never again take LSD.[2]

What is this LSD experience which can give one person a feeling of complete fulfillment, while for another it is "a glimpse into the echoing terror that is insanity"?

What, to begin with, is LSD?

LSD-25 is the laboratory nickname given to the formidably titled indole, d-lysergic acid-diethylamide tartrate, 25. This compound is derived from ergot, which in turn is derived from a black fungus that sometimes develops in rye and other grasses.

During the Middle Ages this black fungus was responsible for epidemics of Saint Anthony's Fire, a disease which caused two kinds of poisoning. In one, arms and legs would first turn blue, then become gangrenous, and ultimately crumble away.[3] The other kind of poisoning began with an itching and tingling of the skin, followed by a loss of sensation which sometimes included deafness and dimness of vision. Often severe psychotic disorders developed which culminated in death. These dreadful epidemics were at last brought under control in the nineteenth century, although rare single cases still appear in medical literature.[4]

Somewhere along the way it was discovered that the black fungus responsible for Saint Anthony's Fire contained a valuable drug, ergot (which is used in difficult pregnancies even today). It is interesting to remember that another fungus was recently discovered to contain the valuable drug, penicillin. A derivative of ergot proved helpful in relieving migraine headaches. A second derivative, lysergic acid, seemed to have no medicinal value and was ignored—until one April afternoon in 1943.

On that day a Swiss chemist, Hoffman, after adding an extra "tail" of a diethylamide group to lysergic acid for the purposes of experimentation, began to feel strange sensations which he later described in a laboratory report:

> I had to give up working because I experienced a very peculiar restlessness which was associated with a slight attack of dizziness. At home I went to bed, and got into a state of not unpleasant drunkenness. . . . When I closed my eyes . . . I experienced fantastic images . . . associated with an intense kaleidoscopic play of colors.[5]

This was the first of all LSD experiences—although Hoffman did not know that. In fact, he did not know what had happened. Puzzling over the episode, he wondered whether he might not accidentally have swallowed or inhaled or ingested through his pores some of the substance with which he had been working. (How many discoveries in science have been accidental? This would be an interesting field of research.)

To test his hypothesis Hoffman deliberately swallowed 25 micrograms of the chemical he had synthesized. After a time, in his words:

> I lost all control of time; space and time became more and more disorganized and I was overcome with fears that I was

going crazy. The worst part of it was that I was clearly aware of my condition though I was incapable of stopping it. Occasionally I felt as being outside my body. I thought I had died. My "Ego" was suspended somewhere in space and I saw my body lying dead on the sofa. I observed and registered clearly that my "alter ego" was moving around the room, moaning.[6]

Hoffman went on to report how certain sounds—an automobile horn, running water, even words—transformed into shapes and colors, a phenomenon known as synesthesia.

Hoffman's experience instigated a series of intensive investigations carried on chiefly by two colleagues, Stoll and Rothlin. After four years of experimentation on volunteer subjects, their findings were published.

According to Stoll and others, the first noticeable changes to appear in the individual under LSD were physiological ones. Pupillary dilation, a deepening and slowing of respiration, tremors, and ataxia occurred regularly. These symptoms were occasionally accompanied by dizziness, headaches, sweating, or mild nausea. Shortly afterwards psychological changes appeared, the most striking of which were visual hallucinations:

> These ranged from prolonged after-images through . . . geometric patterns of varying descriptions and color, to distorted, often grotesque objects such as peacock feathers, Buddhas, and in the case of a chemist, benzol rings. Synesthetic reactions occurred frequently. Sudden auditory stimulation evoked immediate changes in visual phenomena which were reminiscent of Disney's Fantasia. . . .[7]

Remarkably, during these hallucinations, the subject remained lucid and his orientation in space was intact. However his sense of *time* became distorted: time slowed down, or accelerated—or seemed even to be abolished.

This report triggered an epidemic of research into LSD. Since the publication of Stoll's article in 1947, well over six hundred articles on LSD-25 have appeared in the journals of Canada, Hungary, France, South Africa, Italy, Argentina, England, the

United States. Even the Soviet Union in its *Journal of Neurology and Psychiatry* has published an article titled "The Experimental Psychosis and Psychiatric Use of LSD," essentially a digest of the foreign literature.[8]

Out of this welter of experimentation, it is possible to discern two main avenues of research. These are described by Dr. Rinkel and his associates of Boston Hospital, pioneers of LSD exploration in the United States:

> The investigation of the LSD-induced psychosis has brought to light facts which led us to *a new chemical concept of the cause and nature of mental illness.* . . .
>
> (Also) many subjects who had taken the drug, and under its influence experienced mental changes and alterations in behavior, *became more aware of their own problems, which resulted in better adjustment.*[9]

Chiefly, then, LSD research is trying to determine whether or not mental illness can result from chemical changes in the body and, secondly, whether or not LSD can facilitate psychotherapy.

To consider the first question first: how can LSD help to prove that mental illness results from chemical imbalances in the body? Dr. Cholden clarifies this point:

> Let us consider for a moment [he writes] of an ideal tool to help us understand the state of being called schizophrenia. This ideal tool might well be the artificial production of the disease. It must be safe, so that it will not hurt a volunteer; it might reproduce schizophrenia exactly; it might be short-acting; it might be controllable so that we may study the partial effects; it must be reproducible, so that the effects can be checked; and lastly, this tool must allow the subject of the experiment to communicate subjective data to the investigator.[10]

Dr. Cholden suggests that LSD might be such an ideal tool. So do other scientists. As a result, much research was generated in an attempt to understand how LSD affects the mind-body, both chemically and psychologically.

Apparently, with the exceptions of pupillary dilation and ataxia, the physiological changes which occur are inconsistent. Some research workers report an increase in blood pressure and pulse rate under LSD, others a decrease, while still others state that there are no changes in either. Respiratory changes have been described as increased, decreased, and remaining constant. Changes in body temperature have been reported as ranging from feelings of cold with actual chills, to feelings of warmth accompanied by fever, to no change in temperature at all. Visual changes are described as blurred, dimmed, or heightened. (In one instance, vision was reported so heightened that a subject was able to read a newspaper at thirty feet.) Body sensations are described as ranging along one continuum from a tingling of the skin to intense pain in which "the individual's entire being is centered in the painful organ"; and along a second continuum ranging from a loss of sensation in one or another section of the body, to feelings of being transported completely outside one's body, a state described as depersonalization. Changes in the electro-encephalogram are generally reported as minimal—but even these minimal changes are reported variously. One research stated that the Alpha rhythm was blocked under LSD, another stated that the Alpha rhythm was increased, and a third research has reported that out of 22 subjects given LSD, the Alpha rhythm decreased 30 per cent in 11 subjects, increased 50 per cent in 7 subjects, and remained the same in 4 subjects. On a physiological basis, then, there seems to be no indication as to the cause of the LSD "model psychosis" yet.

In the field of biochemistry the findings are more provocative.

It is a challenging fact that although the LSD psychosis lasts eight hours and more, usually, most of the LSD disappears from the body *within one hour after it is ingested,* and it disappears from the brain and bloodstream *within twenty to thirty minutes.* Moreover, one group of scientists, experimenting with cats and monkeys, found that *only 1 per cent* of the LSD ingested was excreted in urine or feces. Apparently the drug undergoes almost a complete metabolic change in the body. Interestingly, Hoagland and others state that LSD in normal subjects causes urinary phosphates which are similar to the urinary phosphates *of schizophrenic patients who have not taken the drug.* Hoffer and Osmond offer similar evidence.

Is schizophrenia, then, caused by a chemical change in the body? And if so, what is the specific chemical change?

Three hypotheses have so far been advanced. One, that LSD creates a model psychosis because of a deficiency in serotonin, · has already been more or less disproved. A second hypothesis states that schizophrenia is caused by a deficiency of acetylcholine.

At the first World Conference of Psychiatry held in Paris in 1950, evidence was submitted to support this statement, and furthermore it was reported that Fiamberti effected successful treatment of schizophrenics by massive parenteral injections of acetylcholine.

Since LSD is a drug which inhibits the production of acetylcholine, further research in support of this hypothesis is indicated but has not as yet been reported.

The third and perhaps most provocative hypothesis suggests that psychosis is related to an involvement of the adrenalin cycle. In the United States, Rinkel and his associates have offered interesting evidence in support of this claim. At approximately the same time, in Canada, Osmond and his associates happened on the same adrenalin hypothesis by an odd chance. One day after playing a tape recording of an LSD session for a professor of history, they were startled to learn that the professor had experienced reactions very similar to those produced by LSD—after he had taken epinephrine (adrenalin) for an asthmatic condition. The professor reported a further curious fact: that his reactions had been most intense when the adrenalin solution had turned pinkish in color. With this information as a clue, Hoffer and Osmond went on to find other instances of people who had experienced LSD-like reactions after taking adrenalin, and again they discovered that the adrenalin reactions had been most intense when the solution had turned pink. By experiment it was determined that the change in color was due to an increased adrenochrome content. (Adrenochrome and adrenolutin are two by-products of adrenalin.)

In a further experiment, Hoffer and Osmond gave LSD to twelve normal subjects—whose mean adrenochrome content rose from an average of 44 to 105. Moreover, the adrenochrome reached its maximum level *at the same time* that the LSD experience, complete with hallucinations, was at its height. These facts suggested that adrenochrome might be the first substance occurring naturally in the body to be an hallucinogen. (All other known substances which cause hallucinations have been derived from plants.)

To test this new supposition, Hoffer and Osmond administered adrenochrome to normal subjects. Within an hour, these subjects developed marked changes in visual perception, delusions, and depressions sometimes tinged with paranoia: reactions typically found in schizophrenics.

Further exploration is needed, of course. And it is being conducted, today, in an attempt to prove that mental illness may be caused by a specific chemical change in the body.

This would be a remarkable result, surely. And one which, even more remarkably, was predicted by the two great pioneers of psychotherapy. Carl Jung stated in 1956:

> Inasmuch as we have been unable to discover any psychologically understandable process to account for the schizophrenic complex, I draw the conclusion that there might be a *toxic* cause. That is, a physiological change has taken place, because the brain cells were subject to emotional stress beyond their capacity. I suggest that here is an almost unexplored region, ready for pioneer research work.[11]

And in 1940, discussing psychoanalytic therapy, Freud wrote:

> We are here concerned with therapy only insofar as it works by psychological methods: and for the time being we have no

other. The future may teach us how to exercise a direct influence by means of *particular chemical substances;* upon the
amounts of energy and their distribution in the apparatus of
the mind. It may be that there are undreamed-of possibilities
of therapy.[12]

"It may be that there are undreamed-of possibilities of
therapy. . . ." Several psychotherapists today believe that LSD
offers one such possibility: on the face of it, a paradox. After
all, to induce an LSD model psychosis in a patient who is already mentally ill, as one doctor remarked, "may sound like
carrying the idea of 'the hair of the dog that bit you' rather
far—but it seems to be justified." [13]

How is it justified? In 1954, Dr. Sandison of Powick Hospital,
England, reported in a medical journal that he had treated 36
mental patients with LSD therapy, and that 27 of them were
either cured or greatly improved. Unequivocally it is stated:

> All of these patients were either severe obsessional neurotics
> with a bad prognosis or were patients who had been ill for a
> considerable time and who had had prolonged treatment either
> by psychotherapy or other means *without improvement.* . . .
> We would stress that we regard all our cases as being very diffi-
> cult psychiatric problems, and that they were all in danger of
> becoming permanent mental invalids, lifelong neurotics, or of
> ending their lives by suicide.[14]

Three years later Sandison and his colleagues reported on
the progress of those original 36 patients. Not only had there
been a low relapse rate, but:

> It should be pointed out that 27 out of the original 36 patients
> required mental hospital in-patient treatment when we first
> saw them, and at the time of writing, as far as we are aware
> (excluding 4 cases inadequately followed up), not one of these
> patients is in a mental hospital.[15]

This data is enriched by a discussion of many additional
cases, totally 96 in all. Out of this group, 65 per cent had either
recovered or were greatly improved; 12 per cent had failed to

respond; and the rest had achieved varying degrees of improvement. Again:

> We must emphasize again the fact that all our earlier cases and
> most of the later ones had failed to respond to conventional
> methods of therapy.[16]

The article goes on to describe the therapeutic technique employed with LSD. Exploratory interviews are conducted two weeks before the drug is administered. Then the patient is given an LSD session once a week for eight to ten weeks, longer if necessary. A typical session lasts from five to eight hours, during which time the patient is under constant supervision either by a nurse or by the therapist in charge.

According to Sandison, LSD evokes manifestations of the "psychic unconscious" which generally fall into one of two categories. In the first, hallucinations—or fantasies—develop, which the patient experiences with extraordinary intensity and reality. Such fantasies, according to these doctors, are invaluable for therapy:

> Just as dreams have come to be regarded as a source of material for Freudian and Jungian analysis, so the experiences of the patients under LSD might be similarly used.[17]

Again and again the patient recognizes one of these fantasies to be a symbol of a real life conflict. This is possible because, throughout the hallucination, the patient's consciousness is not impaired: the patient is able to interpret his dreams, even as he participates in them. Often the very recognition of such a fantasy symbol leads to a resolution of the patient's problem either during the session itself, or in later interviews when the material is discussed and evaluated. The significance of LSD hallucinations has been overlooked by many investigators, Sandison suggests, first because the physiological symptoms have been a primary consideration and secondly because

> the random observations of normal subjects under LSD appear
> confused, disintegrated, and haphazard compared with the

much more orderly train of events which occur in patients undergoing LSD treatment. This is probably because the patient is under the control of the therapist where he is taught to concentrate upon each image as it appears and to follow it to its conclusion.[18]

As an example of a fantasy that has therapeutic value, the hallucination of one patient is described, in which she saw two women:

> . . . one [was] a middle-aged, large, coarse woman dressed in an unpleasant and untidy purple dress, and having a revolting smell. The other was a beautiful woman dressed in the style of the French court before the Revolution. She alternately became both of these women. . . .
> This experience agreed well with her biographical details and helped her greatly to understand her position.[19]

Another example of an hallucination which was of much therapeutic value is described, in the patient's own words, in a report she made after having been given an LSD session at a time she was in deep depression and on the point of suicide:

> I had the sensation . . . of a snake curling up around me . . . I then began to see serpents' faces all over the wall—then I saw myself as a fat, pot-bellied snake slithering gaily away to destruction. I felt horrified and thought, "Whose destruction?" I then realized it was my own destruction—I was destroying myself. I seemed to be having a battle between life and death —it was a terrific struggle, but life won. I then saw myself on the treadmill of life—a huge wheel was going round and round with hundreds of people on it. Some were on top going confidently through life, others were getting jostled and trodden on but still struggling to go on living (I saw myself as one of these people) and then there were the others who just couldn't cope with life and were being crushed to death in the wheel. I had another realization of how I was destroying myself—by carrying on this affair with this married man. . . . I knew it must cease and knew that I must never see him again.[20]

A second major advantage of LSD therapy, according to Sandison and his colleagues, is the emergence of early traumas which the patient has totally forgotten. This is *not* a mere remembrance of the incident. Rather, it is a *re-experiencing:* the patient feels himself becoming a child, or even a baby, and the patient by voice, gesture, and manner acts like the child he has been and feels the emotions he had felt originally. This is a phenomenon known as "abreaction." Sandison declares that the abreactions produced under LSD are the "most intense" he has ever seen, and offers as an example the woman patient who felt herself, under LSD, transforming into a little girl:

> She felt that her clothes were huge and hung loosely about her, and when the doctor grasped her hand, his hand seemed large as an adult's hand would seem to a child. In a series of experiences accompanied by intense emotion, she relived sexual assaults on her by a man during her childhood. She described a wood near her home where one of the incidents had taken place, even seeing the floor (of the hospital room) apparently carpeted with wild plants and flowers. At the height of this abreaction, she told how the man repeatedly threatened to kill her if she told anyone about the occurrence.[21]

The patient had repressed this experience from her conscious mind completely. However the memory had remained with her, unconsciously, and had expressed itself in the form of a severe neurosis

> in which the patient had been tortured by all sorts of obsessions regarding water and spent the great part of her life performing washing rituals. . . . Except for a few months after her marriage, she had not been free of these symptoms since the age of thirteen. At her worst, she was at times suicidal; at other times, she was confined to bed, or spent up to eight hours a day washing herself, or her own and her child's clothes.[22]

This patient, who had not responded to any other form of treatment, was cured by LSD therapy, and has remained well.

Sandison and his colleagues further believe that LSD considerably shortens the therapeutic process:

> Early LSD experiences frequently lead one straight to the core of the patient's problem. They do so more surely and more frequently than is normal in psychotherapy and many months of time can be saved. I am convinced that patients under LSD come to the central problem long before they can possibly realize it by ordinary analytic means . . .[23]

Far from decrying the psychoanalytic theories,

> If anyone wants confirmation of the great analytic principles laid down by Freud and Jung, let him study patients having LSD.[24]

The first of these articles on LSD therapy appeared in an English journal in 1954. The following year a German scientist, Frederking, published an article in a German journal, stating that he had been using LSD in therapy for three years, and mescalin (another hallucinogen) for seventeen years. Frederking describes the hallucinations produced by these drugs as "waking dreams" and believes, like Sandison, that they can be as meaningful for therapy as the dreams dreamed at night which are brought in to the therapist for interpretation. Again like Sandison, Frederking reports that under LSD childhood memories emerge which are relived with intense emotion, producing an abreaction of much therapeutic value. As illustration, Frederking gives the case history of a twenty-five-year-old man who had chronically suffered from impotence. This patient had been in psychoanalysis for a considerable time, and had often mentioned that he was highly sensitive around the navel—a condition which he was at a loss to explain. Given his first LSD session the patient regressed to

> a small, helpless child subject to titillation of the navel and genitalia, and other kinds of torture. [Later] upon questioning his mother we found that for several months, in the first half of his second year, he had had much to suffer at the hands of a nurse.[25]

The nurse had of course been discharged—but not before she had damaged the patient, almost irretrievably. Several LSD sessions, however, relieved the patient of his impotence.

Gradually, psychotherapists of many countries began to explore the possibilities of LSD in therapy. Reports of these findings have been published in the medical journals of Italy, Canada, South Africa, England, the United States, Argentina and other countries. (See Bibliography.) Majority opinion, as expressed in these articles, concurs with Sandison and Frederking that LSD is a useful adjunct to psychotherapy. There are, nevertheless, minority reports. One article claims that the LSD reaction can be too stunning and may shatter the patient's necessary defenses. Another objection is that the benefits of LSD therapy may not be permanent. A second article straddles the issue, stating that the release of repressed emotions can be therapeutic at times, though at other times it is not. At the end of this continuum there is a report which states that LSD is of no therapeutic value in mental illness. But overall, it is urged that LSD offers a striking advantage in the treatment of the psychoneuroses.

LSD therapy has been extended to include alcoholics, with encouraging results. One article reports on a group of 24 chronic alcoholics (all but four of whom had tried Alcoholics Anonymous and failed), who were given LSD therapy. Twelve of these seemingly hopeless cases were described as either improved, or much improved. Unfortunately, there is no report on the permanence of the treatment. In another report of LSD therapy with alcoholics, the cure would seem to have been of a temporary nature.

Going beyond the neuroses into the darker region of schizophrenia, there have been a few interesting experiments. Cholden and his colleagues report the following incident of a psychotic patient who had been given LSD:

> One catatonic patient who had been mute for some years suddenly burst into loud wailing sobs which were shortly followed by overwhelming bursts of laughter. . . . Intermittently she

would open her mouth as if she were trying desperately to talk.
. . . She also expressed a state of acute anguish in her body
movements. When asked why she had been crying, she said:
"You should never leave the farm. . . ."

That evening she went to a dance and danced with another
patient for the first time. She continued talking until bedtime.
The next morning when she woke, she was her old catatonic
self.[26]

What quality in the drug LSD made this woman speak and
participate socially for the first time in years? No one yet knows.
But research goes on.

Apart from psychotherapy and psychosis, exploration of LSD
is being urged for other purposes. Eisner and Cohen state that

for the therapist, researcher, and individual interested in human dynamics, LSD is extraordinary, if only because of the
rich view of the unconscious which it permits.[27]

Somewhere in this rich view of the unconscious lies the mystic
experience described by Aldous Huxley. Certain investigators
believe this to be an important area of research, and suggest
that the amazing vistas which open to the individual under
LSD need not be considered hallucinations. Stevenson, for
example, argues that the music, colors, and objects which a
person under LSD perceives do not change. Rather something
within the person changes. But what is it that changes?

If I put on glasses and see details more clearly, no one can
say that I am hallucinating. But if, under the drug, I see colors
and forms I did not see before, they say I am hallucinating.
But maybe I really have achieved a new and better vision of
external reality. . . .

These drugs may bring us at least partially into a world of
which we know little and should know a great deal more.[28]

Leaving the antipodes of mysticism for a far sterner outpost,
it has been suggested that LSD might prove an effective—because harmless—means of chemical warfare, for the drug creates

a psychosis which only temporarily incapacitates the individual from normal functioning.

The most recent LSD explorations have appeared—in the most unlikely of places—at a cancer symposium held in Kentucky in 1960. After ten years of experimentation with tumors in animals, Dr. Scott of the University of California reported that he had discovered a chemical which was effective in blocking cancerous growths in animals. "Strangely enough," writes the Los Angeles *Times* of March 27, 1960, "the chemical is LSD-25, the hallucination-producing drug used by psychiatrists to simulate mental illness."

In view of the wide range of possible applications for LSD, Sandison's metaphor, derived from an English novel, seems well chosen. In the book, a "magical stone" is recovered after having been lost for many centuries.

"Some people used this magical stone as a means of transportation, some used it as a means of healing, some used it as a means of gaining philosophical insight into the world's problems, and some used it as a means of gaining political power." [29]

LSD may eventually be used for one (or all?) of these purposes.

APPENDIX B:

Reality versus Psychic Reality

FREUD began practice in Vienna as a specialist in nervous diseases. One such disease was hysteria, at the time considered virtually incurable.

However, Breuer, colleague and mentor, described to Freud how he had cured a patient of hysteria, using hypnosis as his major therapeutic device. Freud soon began to apply Breuer's method to his own patients. Over a period of years, he came to discard hypnosis altogether, for he had evolved a new kind of therapeutic technique which he called psychoanalysis.

In 1896 he published a paper, claiming to have *cured* thirteen cases of the "virtually incurable" hysteria. Moreover, Freud stated that in all thirteen cases, the "hysterical symptoms are traced to their origin which invariably proves to be an experience in the person's sexual life . . . either . . . a brutal attempt committed by an adult . . . or a less sudden and repugnant seduction, having however the same result." [1]

At this midday of Victorian morality this was an outrageous statement—outrageous, it would seem, to Freud himself:

> How can one be convinced of the truth of these confessions made in analysis and said to be memories preserved since early childhood, and how can we protect ourselves against the inclination to fabricate and the facility for invention ascribed to hysterics? I would charge myself with blameworthy credulity if I did not offer more convincing proofs. But the fact is that

the patients never relate these histories spontaneously, and never suddenly offer, in the course of the treatment, the complete recollection of such a scene to the physician. The mental image of a premature sexual experience is recalled only . . . against strong resistance. [In my LSD experience, I had battled fierce resistance before arriving at the mental image of myself as a little girl being forced to lie down, and then raped.] If we . . . are able to follow impartially, in detail, the psychoanalysis of a case of hysteria, we are finally convinced ourselves.[2]

Freud was *not* "finally convinced" because the very next year in a letter to his great friend, Wilhelm Fliess:

Let me tell you straight away the great secret which has been slowly dawning on me in recent months. *I no longer believe in my neurotica.* . . . There was the astonishing fact that *in every case* . . . blame was laid on perverse acts by the father, though it was hardly credible that perverse acts against children were so general. . . . [Also] there was the definite realization that there is no "indication of reality" in the unconscious, so that it is important to distinguish between truth and emotionally-charged fiction. . . . Now I do not know where I am. . . . Can these doubts be only an episode on the way to further knowledge?[3]

Freud was kept "on the way to further knowledge" by these doubts for several years:

It is not surprising that during ten years of constant work towards elucidating these problems, I should have travelled some distance beyond my previous point of view. . . . I was not at this period able to discriminate between the deceptive memories of hysterics concerning their childhood and the memory traces of actual happenings.[4]

Deceptive memories and *memory traces of actual happenings.* Here were the seeds of *psychic reality* and *reality*, not yet formulated into a concept. These ten years were extremely difficult ones for Freud. Looking back at them he wrote these candid words:

One was easily inclined to regard as real . . . the accounts of patients who traced back their symptoms to passive sexual occurrences in the first years of their childhood—speaking frankly, to seductions. When this etiology broke down through its own unlikelihood . . . there followed a period of absolute helplessness. The analysis had led . . . to such infantile sexual traumas, and yet, these were not true. Thus, the basis of *reality* had been lost. At that time, I would gladly have dropped the whole thing. . . . Perhaps I persevered only because I had no longer any choice of beginning something else. Finally, I reflected that after all no one has a right to despair if he has been disappointed in his expectations; one must merely revise them. If hysterics trace back their symptoms to imaginary traumas, then this new fact signifies that they create such scenes *in fantasy*, and hence *psychic reality deserves to be given a place next to actual reality.*[5]

At this juncture, in 1914, Freud had given psychic reality a place next to actual reality, presumably an inferior place.

Three years later, he revised this concept. In one of his *Introductory Lectures*, Freud describes how his patients in analysis revealed scenes of infantile seduction. . . .

Now the astonishing thing is that these scenes of infancy are not always true. . . . This discovery is more likely than any other to discredit . . . the analysis. . . . There is, besides this, something utterly bewildering about it. If the infantile experiences brought to light by the analysis were in every case real, we should have the feeling we were on firm ground; if they were invariably falsified and found to be inventions and fantasies of the patient, we should have to forsake this insecure foothold and save ourselves some other way. *But it is neither one thing nor the other:* for what we find is that the childhood experiences reconstructed or recollected are on some occasions undeniably false, while others are just as certainly quite true, and that in most cases, *truth and falsehood are mixed up.* . . . It is hard to find one's way here. . . . We are tempted to be offended with the patient for taking up our time with invented stories. . . . The patient himself, incidentally, takes this same attitude [of impatience with the therapist]. It takes him a long time to understand the proposal that fantasy and reality are to be treated alike and that it is to begin with of no account whether the childhood experience under consideration belongs to one class or the other. . . . It is a fact that the patient has created these fantasies, and for the neurosis this fact is hardly less important than the other. . . . In contrast to material *reality* these fantasies possess *psychic reality* and we gradually come to understand that *in the world of neurosis, psychic reality is the determining factor.*[6]

Freud had now given *psychic reality* the edge over reality. Ultimately, he was to say:

The majority of my patients reproduced from their childhood scenes in which they were sexually seduced by some grownup person. With female patients, the part of the seducer was almost always assigned to the father. I believed these stories, and consequently supposed that I had discovered the roots of the subsequent neurosis in these experiences of sexual seductions in childhood. . . . If the reader feels inclined to shake his head at my credulity, I cannot altogether blame him; though I may plead that this was at a time when I was intentionally keeping my critical faculties in abeyance so as to preserve an unprejudiced and receptive attitude towards the many novelties that were coming to my attention every day. When, however, I was at last obliged to recognize that these scenes of seduction had never taken place, and that they were only fantasies which my patients had made up . . . I was for some time completely at a loss. . . . When I had pulled myself together, I was able to draw the right conclusions from my discovery: namely, that the neurotic symptoms were not directly related to actual events but to fantasies embodying wishes, and that as far as the neurosis was concerned, psychic reality was *of more importance* than material reality.[7]

Freud then was finally convinced that psychic reality was more important than reality in the understanding of neurosis. He arrived at this conviction after more than twenty years of exploration, bewilderment, and revisions in his thinking.

APPENDIX C:

Displacement

W HEN Jack gets married "on the rebound," we infer that Jack is trying to transfer the love he felt for one woman to another. This transfer of emotion is called, in psychiatric terms, "displacement." Love can be displaced, or hate, or any other emotion. Not only can emotions be displaced from person to person, but also from person to thing: "When Bismarck had to suppress his angry feelings in the King's presence, he relieved himself afterwards by smashing a valuable vase on the floor." [1]

There are myriad displacements in our lives, some of them so persistent that they form a lifetime pattern of behavior: "That the lonely spinster transfers her affection to animals, that the bachelor becomes a passionate collector, that the soldier defends a scrap of colored cloth—his flag—with his life blood, that in a love affair a clasp of the hands a moment longer than usual evokes a sensation of bliss, or that in Othello a lost handkerchief causes an outburst of rage—all these are examples of psychic displacements." [2]

Rebound marriages, barroom belligerencies, spilled-milk tantrums, and similar phenomena have been recognized for hundreds of years. But it was Freud who organized these various, isolated behaviors into one general principle which he called displacement.

Freud stressed the fact that displacement is more often than not an unconscious process.

In recent years, trying to demonstrate this hypothesis empirically, scientists have devised controlled experiments with such diverse subjects as rats, children, monkeys, and men. Several of these experiments have offered striking corroboration of Freud's postulate. For example:

It was found that a child would not show her anger to a parent—but she would afterwards spank her doll savagely. This presents a triangle very similar to the vase, the king, and Bismarck. It was also shown that the *amount* of overt anger increases, inversely, with the *distance* of displacement. That is to say, a child shows almost no anger toward a parent; some toward a teacher; more toward a brother or sister; and most against a doll or toy. Apparently, the less dangerous the situation, the more emotion expressed.

Even rats have been shown to utilize displacement in their behavior. In one experiment, Rat A was trained to avoid a painful shock by hitting at Rat B with his paw. Then Rat B was taken away, and a doll substituted for him. Rat A, to avoid the shock, hit at the doll with his paw in just the way he had hit at Rat B. Here the displacement was from an animal to an object.[3]

Displacement, then, seems to be a universal phenomenon—and probably a necessary one. If as babies we did not learn to displace our need/desire for the nipple of the breast to the nipple of the bottle to the rim of a cup or glass, we would be in a fine fix, surely. And if we did not displace our love for the immediate members of the family to other members of society, then society would find itself in a fine fix.

Freud discovered that displacement was particularly evident in dreams. He pointed out that simple dreams are no more than undisguised wish fulfillments:

A little girl nineteen months old had been kept without food all day because she had had an attack of vomiting in the morning: her nurse declared that she had been upset by eating strawberries. During the night after this day of starvation, she was heard saying her own name in her sleep and adding "Stwaw-bewwies, wild stwawbewwies, omblet, pap!" She was thus dream-ing of eating a meal and she laid special stress in her menu on the particular delicacy of which, she had reason to expect, she would only be allowed scanty quantities in the near future.[4]

But not many of our dreams are so simple and undisguised. Often our wishes are so repulsive to us that even in our dreams we disguise them. And to disguise them, we use, unconsciously of course, this mechanism of displacement: We shift the wish we feel regarding one person to another person, or to a con-glomerate person, or to a thing. As a result, we wake up from such a dream thinking that it was confused and meaningless. This is a most difficult concept to understand—or accept.

How could a dream such as the one I had had about my very fat aunt—with only half her body—be the expression of a *wish?* I did not believe it could be. Until one day, in fantasy, I saw a long brown skirt covering my mother's very fat (very preg-nant) stomach. That image so infuriated me that I began to hack at her stomach to destroy the foetus—and found myself back in the nightmare of my very fat aunt who was without the lower half of her body.

Instead of dreaming about my mother without the lower half of her body, and hence without the foetus I wished to de-stroy, I had substituted my aunt. My murderous wish had been fulfilled in this dream, through the mechanism of displacement.

But why was this displacement necessary? Why did I not simply dream of my mother without her pregnant stomach?

Because, although I hated my mother for having a new baby, at the same time I loved her and did not wish to hurt her. This simultaneous love/hate created a conflict in me. And "the child finds relief from the conflict . . . by displacing his hostile and fearful feelings on to a substitute."[5]

It might be argued—I argued it myself—that as a child of two and a half, I could not have known that my mother was pregnant with my sister. Presumably I had no idea, then, where babies come from. This notion is here disabused:

> Lately, by the analysis of a five year old boy . . . I have received an irrefutable proof of a piece of knowledge toward which the psychoanalysis of adults had for a long time led me. I now know that the changes in the mother during pregnancy do not escape the sharp eyes of a child, and that the latter is very well able subsequently to establish the correct connection between the increase in size of the mother's body and the appearance of a baby. In the case mentioned, the boy was three and a half when his sister was born, and four and three quarters when he showed his better knowledge by the most unmistakable allusions. This precocious knowledge is however . . . repressed and forgotten.[6]

APPENDIX D:

Puns and Word Play

As WE have seen in Appendix C, one major process of the unconscious, according to Freud, is displacement. Another major process of the unconscious, again according to Freud, is "condensation," which "strives to condense two different thoughts by selecting, *after the manner of wit,* an ambiguous word which can suggest both thoughts." [1]

Also: "A name is made use of twice: first as a whole and then divided into its syllables and in their divided state the syllables yield a different meaning." [2]

We have already had a superb example of this unconscious process called condensation by Freud in my LSD image of the Peapod. After the manner of wit, this ambiguous word suggested two different thoughts which became apparent when the word Peapod was divided into its syllables: *pea* which yields the meaning of urine; and *pod* which means something that contains seeds. These two different thoughts combine to form out of the word "peapod," a synomym for the penis, an instrument which combines the two functions of emitting urine, and also seeds.

This kind of word play, or pun, is far from an isolated phenomenon in dreams or fantasies or free association. In fact, so many "comical and bizarre word formations" popped up in Freud's investigations that he was impelled to make a study of the principles of humor which he published in a book called *Wit and Its Relation to the Unconscious.*

In this work, Freud first describes the process of condensation as it is found in conscious humor such as puns or word plays or jokes.

One such example, offered by Brill: "Disraeli once remarked that old persons are apt to fall into 'anecdotage.' . . . On analysis we find that [anecdotage] is made up of two words, anecdote and dotage. . . . Disraeli fuses the two words into a neologism, anecdotage, and thus simultaneously expresses both ideas. Such a fusion of words is called *condensation*." [3]

Another, similar example taken from literature (again reported by Brill): "In a short story which I have recently read, one of the characters, a 'sport,' speaks of the Christmas season as the *alcoholidays*." [4] *Alcohol* and *holidays* combine to create this amusing condensation.

Condensation also occurs in "double meaning with ambiguity," which frequently forms the basis of joke humor. Freud gives this joke as an instance:

> [There is] the story told of a wealthy but elderly gentleman who showed his devotion to a young actress by many lavish gifts. Being a respectable girl, she took the first opportunity to discourage his attentions by telling him that her heart was already given to another man. "I never aspired as high as that," was his polite answer.[5]

Such "double meaning with ambiguity" appears not only in the conscious humor of jokes, but also in the quite unconscious process of dreams and fantasies. Freud gives as an instance a short dream related by a patient: "*His uncle gives him a kiss in an auto.* He [the patient] immediately adds the interpretation, which would never have occurred to me; it means *auto-erotism*." [6]

Freud then goes on to give another, more complex illustration—at his own expense:

> A skeptical patient had a dream "in which certain people were telling her about my book on Wit and praising it very highly."

> Then something else came in about a canal . . . *something to do with a canal . . . it was quite vague. . . .*

The dreamer had no association to the word *canal;* naturally I did not know what to say either. Shortly afterwards she told me that an association had occurred to her which *perhaps* had something to do with it. It was, in fact, a witty remark which someone had told her. On board ship between Dover and Calais, a well-known author was talking to an Englishman who in some particular context quoted the words: "Du sublime au ridicule il n'y a qu'un *pas.*" (It's only a *step* from the sublime to the ridiculous.) The author answered: "Oui, Le *Pas* de Calais," meaning that he regarded France as sublime and England as ridiculous. Of course the *Pas* de Calais is a *canal*—that is to say, Canal La Manche—the English Channel. Now, you ask, do I think this association has anything to do with the dream? Certainly I think so. . . . The association reveals the skepticism disguised under the obtrusive admiration.[7]

Freud recognized that dream puns and word plays such as these seem deliberately contrived: they are almost *too* witty. But so many of them appeared so often in his years of practice that he eventually postulated the process of condensation as a definite unconscious mechanism.

Subsequent investigations, by psychiatrists and psychologists as well as psychoanalysts, corroborate his postulate. Very recently a clinical psychologist reported a brief dream of a patient who was about to go on a trip to an unknown destination by means of a ship named the *Newland.* The therapist inferred from this fragment that the patient had reached a turning point in her therapy and was going to improve. This prophecy (which proved to be correct) was based solely on the name of the ship which the patient had seen in the dream, the *Newland.* Separating this ambiguous word into its syllables we discover that the patient is embarking for a *new land.*

Another example, from a recent group-therapy experience: One of the patients arrived late to a session and explained that she had been detained by an unexpected visit from her father whom she described as a "pill," with some distaste. After leaving him and en route to the session, she had been forced to stop because of an attack of diarrhea. The patient was asked what kind of "pill" her father was. She smiled as if the question were irrelevant and silly, and replied that he was no particular kind of pill: she was just using a colloquial expression. She was then asked if the "pill" might be a laxative. Her involuntary reply was "No!" But then she laughed and said: "Well . . . maybe. After all, I did have that attack of diarrhea after I left father. . . ."

One last, rather poetic illustration: *The dreamer sees three lions in a desert, one of which is laughing, but she is not afraid of them.*

> The analysis yields the following material: The indifferent occasion of the dream was a sentence in the dreamer's English exercise: "The *lion*'s greatest adornment is his mane." Her father used to wear a beard which encircled his face like a *mane.* The name of her English teacher is Miss *Lyons.* An acquaintance of hers had sent her the ballads of *Loewe* (*Loewe* = lion). These, then, are the three lions; why should she be afraid of them? . . . Then followed fragmentary recollections in the merriest mood, such as the following directions for catching lions (from *Die Fliegende Blatter*): "Take a desert and put it through a sieve; the lions will be left behind." . . . The whole matter becomes intelligible as soon as one learns that on the dream day the lady had received a visit from her husband's superior. He was very polite to her and kissed her hand and *she was not at all afraid of him,* although he . . . plays the part of a *"social lion"* in the capital of her country. This lion is, therefore, like the lion in *A Midsummer Night's Dream,* who is unmasked as Snug the Joiner: and of such stuff are all the dream-lions of which one is not afraid.[8]

APPENDIX E:

The Trauma

To CLARIFY the following, I will use as illustration my own childhood trauma: the too strong, too hot enema.

Toward the end of the Christmas season of 1895-96, Freud sent to his friend Wilhelm Fliess a treatise called: *DRAFT K, The Neuroses of Defense (A Christmas Fairy Tale).* In his "Fairy Tale," Freud for the first time postulated that hysteria—believed to be an hereditary illness—might originate in an "overwhelming of the ego" at an early age.

> The increase of tension is so great . . . that the ego does not resist it and constructs no physical symptom, but is obliged to allow a manifestation of discharge to occur—usually an excessive expression of excitation. This first stage of hysteria may be described as "fright hysteria": its primary symptom is a manifestation of *fright* accompanied by a *gap* in the psyche. It is still unknown up to how late an age the first hysterical overwhelming of the ego can take place. Repression and formation of defensive symptoms can only occur afterwards, in connection with the memory.[1]

Miss Leahy's enema had so overwhelmed my ego that when I approached this repressed memory in therapy, I responded with "screams and screams and screams of bull terror *in a void*." This would be the first stage of hysteria, according to Freud: "a *fright* hysteria, accompanied by a *gap* in the psyche."

Not a year later, Freud published a scientific paper: "The Defense Neuro-Psychoses." After repeating his fairy tale notion about a trauma precipitating hysteria, Freud hazards the years during which such an "overwhelming of the ego" may occur: years so very young that Freud can not hide his own disbelief:

> The lower limit extends as far as memory itself, that is, therefore, to the tender age of from one and a half to two years! (Two cases.) In a number of my cases the sexual trauma (or series of traumas) occurred in the third or fourth year. I should not myself give credence to these singular revelations if they had not proved worthy of belief by the part they played in the subsequent development of the neurosis.[2]

Four years later, Freud seems to have displaced his own disbelief on to the public:

> It is painful to me to think that many of the hypotheses upon which I base my psychological solutions of the psychoneuroses will arouse skepticism and ridicule when they first become known. For instance, I shall have to assert that impressions from the second year of life, and even the first, leave an enduring trace upon the emotional life of subsequent neuropaths, and that these impressions—although greatly distorted and exaggerated by memory—may furnish the earliest and profoundest basis of an hysterical symptom. Patients to whom I explain this at a suitable moment are wont to parody my explanation by offering to search for reminiscences of the period *when they were not yet born.*[3]

I could have been such a parodist. Certainly, during my analysis, I denied and ridiculed that an experience in infancy could affect profoundly one's adult behavior. Furthermore, I was convinced that I had never suffered any such experience: if there had been in my early life an incident or trauma *so painful,* then of course I would remember it.

Freud recognized these objections: "It would indeed be quite useless to question an hysteric outside analysis about these traumas of childhood: *their traces are never found in the conscious memory, only in the symptoms of illness.*" [4]

Actually, it had proved useless to question me *inside* analysis. It was only in LSD therapy that the enema trauma revealed itself . . . in a series of symptoms . . . over several weeks' time.

The first symptom to develop was the bothersome itching rash. The second was the terrible tensions in my arms. Next, I wrapped my arms around my body one day and said: "I feel as if I were going to burst or explode . . ." after which I added: "I'm a long scream through the tunnel."

Finally, under LSD, I had the extraordinary experience of my arms flinging themselves crisscross over my chest, as if propelled by some outside force.

These symptoms had occurred, one by one, for weeks *before* I arrived at the denouement: my arms being tied down and being given an enema when I had the chicken pox and measles.

Bearing in mind the episode in which my arms had propelled themselves across my chest in violent motor activity, after which I had seen the image of Miss Leahy, it is interesting to read this excerpt:

> There are also attacks which seem to consist of nothing but *motor* symptoms. . . . If we succeed in summoning up an attack while the patient is under hypnosis [substitute *under LSD*], we find these attacks are based on memories of a psychic trauma or series of traumas which usually finds expression in an hallucinatory phase. For instance, a little girl has suffered for years from attacks of general convulsions which might have been epilepsy and had in fact been taken for it. To establish a differential diagnosis, she was hypnotized and was promptly seized by an attack. When asked "What do you see now?" she answered "The dog, the dog is coming!" Further inquiry revealed that the first attack of the kind had appeared after she had been chased by a mad dog. Therapeutic success later confirmed the diagnosis of a psychogenic malady.[5]

Seeing a mad dog under hypnosis was the little girl's "hallucinatory phase." Seeing a strange nurse whom I called Miss Leahy under LSD would be a similar "hallucinatory phase."

In both cases, therapeutic success confirmed the "psychogenic" nature of the malady.

For many many years Freud explored the traumas of infancy and childhood which were revealed to him by patients. Gradually the hypothesis he had tentatively set forth in his "Christmas Fairy Tale" strengthened into one of his strongest tenets: that events of the first five years profoundly influence one's entire adult behavior:

> When, during the treatment of an adult neurotic, we tried to trace the determination of his symptoms we were always led back to early childhood. . . . We came to see that the first years of infancy (up to about the age of five) are, for a number of reasons, of especial importance. This is . . . because the impressions of this period come up against an unformed and weak ego, upon which they act like traumas. The ego cannot defend itself against the emotional storms which they call forth except by repression, and in this way it acquires in childhood all its predispositions to subsequent illnesses and disturbances of function.[6]

Finally (posthumously), this trenchant statement:

> It seems that neuroses are only acquired during early childhood (up to the age of six), even though their symptoms may not make their appearance until much later. . . . Neuroses are, as we know, disorders of the ego; and it is not to be wondered at that the ego, while it is weak, immature, and incapable of resistance, should fail in dealing with problems which it could later manage with the utmost ease. The helpless ego fends off these problems by attempts at flight (by repressions) which later turn out to be ineffective and which involve permanent hindrances to further development.[7]

My ego would have been able to manage a too-strong enema with the "utmost ease" had it occurred later in life. But at the age of two and a half, my ego was "helpless" and could only fend off the problem—by repression, which later turned out to be ineffective and involved the "permanent hindrance to further development"—of frigidity.

Freud concluded with this provocative metaphor:

> The damage inflicted upon the ego by its first experiences may seem disproportionately great; but we have only to take as an analogy the differences in the effects produced by the prick of a needle upon a mass of germ cells during segmentation . . . and upon the complete animal which develops out of them.[8]

The damage—frigidity—inflicted upon my ego by an early enema seems disproportionately great, certainly. . . . But, using Freud's analogy, the "pinprick" of a too-strong enema on a "segmenting" or developing ego produced a sexually crippled woman, in much the same way that a pinprick into segmenting germ cells will develop some sort of mutation. The same pinprick—a too strong enema—would cause no more concern to my adult ego than would a pinprick trouble the completed animal which develops out of segmenting germ cells.

NOTES AND REFERENCES

CHAPTER 1

1. Thomas Wolfe. *Look Homeward, Angel.*
2. *Sexual Behavior in the Human Female,* 273 ff.

CHAPTER 2

1. *Le Sommeil et Les Rêves.*
2. *Schlaf und Traum.*
3. *Conditioned Reflexes,* 395.
4. *Interpretation of Dreams,* 532.
5. *Journal of Experimental Psychology.* Vol. 3. Pp. 1-14.
6. *New Introductory Lectures,* 104.
7. *Practice of Psychotherapy.* Vol. 16. P. 309.
8. *Collected Papers.* Vol. IV. Pp. 335 ff. Italics mine.
9. *The Question of Lay Analysis,* 33 ff. Italics mine.
10. *New Introductory Lectures,* 104.
11. *The Ego and the Id,* 30.
12. P. 207 ff.

CHAPTER 3

1. P. 14.
2. See Appendix A.
3. Funk and Wagnalls' *College Standard Dictionary.*
4. *Interpretation of Dreams,* 63.
5. *The Archetypes and the Collective Unconscious,* 190. Italics mine.
6. Joseph Breuer and Sigmund Freud, *Studies on Hysteria,* 275 ff.
7. R. A. Sandison, A. M. Spencer, J. D. A. Whitelaw. "The Therapeutic Value of Lysergic Acid Diethylamide in Mental Illness." *The Journal of Mental Science.* Vol. 100. No. 419. P. 497.
8. *Ibid.*
9. *LSD and Mescaline in Experimental Psychiatry.* Louis Cholden, ed. See Bibliography for pertinent individual articles by Abramson, Busch and Johnson, Eisner and Cohen, Lewis and Sloane, and Chandler and Hartman.
10. Sandison and Whitelaw. "Further Studies in the Therapeutic Value of Lysergic Acid Diethylamide in Mental Illness." *Journal of Mental Science.* Vol. 103.
11. Sandison, Spencer, Whitelaw. *Op. Cit.*
12. *Introductory Lectures on Psychoanalysis,* 387. Incidentally, the medical use of

hypnosis was not endorsed by the American Medical Association until 1957. Of further interest concerning hypnosis, Freud wrote: "We psychoanalysts . . . should not forget how much encouragement and theoretical enlightenment we owe to it" (*Collected Papers*, Vol. 5. P. 13).

CHAPTER 5

1. *Collected Papers*. Vol I. P. 316.
2. *Introductory Lectures*, 366.
3. Breuer and Freud. *Studies on Hysteria*. 296 ff.

CHAPTER 7

1. O. Spurgeon English and Gerald H. J. Pearson. *Emotional Problems of Living*, 81.

CHAPTER 8

1. *An Autobigraphical Study*, 62.
2. Pp. 35 ff.

CHAPTER 11

1. This process of displacement was to appear many times in the course of therapy. If the reader is interested to know its *modus operandi*, there is a brief description in Appendix C.
2. P. 481.
3. *Ibid*. P. 244 ff.
4. For some colorful examples of this device, culled from psychological literature, see Appendix D.

CHAPTER 13

1. *The Origins of Psychoanalysis*, 222 ff. Italics mine.
2. *The Interpretation of Dreams*, 32, 33.

CHAPTER 15

1. Freud. *Collected Papers*. Vol. I. Pp. 58, 213.

APPENDIX A

1. Ivan Tors. *Impressions Received After Taking LSD*.
2. Paul Terrell. "I Went Experimentally Insane."
3. Robert De Ropp. *Drugs and the Mind*, 187.
4. *Encyclopedia Britannica*. Vol. 8. P. 683.
5. De Ropp. *Op. Cit*.
6. Charles Savage and Louis Cholden. "Schizophrenia and the Model Psychosis." *Journal of Clinical and Experimental Psychopathology*. Vol. 17. Pp. 405 ff.
7. W. A. Stoll. "Lysergsaure-diathylamid, ein Phantastikum aus der Mutterkorngruppe" in *The Relation of Psychiatry to Pharmacology*, by Abraham Wikler.
8. Oscar Janiger. *Bibliography of LSD Literature*.

9. Max Rinkel. "Biochemical Reflections on the Psychosis Problem" in *LSD and Mescaline*.

10. Louis Cholden. "Introduction" in *LSD and Mescaline*.

11. Voice of America Broadcast. 1956.

12. *An Outline of Psychoanalysis*, 78 ff. Italics mine.

13. Harry Pennes. "Clinical Experiences with New Hallucinations" in *Annals of the New York Academy of Science*, 1957.

14. Sandison, Whitelaw, Spencer. Pp. 491 ff.

15. Sandison and Whitelaw. Pp. 332 ff.

16. *Ibid.*

17. Sandison. "The Clinical Uses of LSD" in *LSD and Mescaline*.

18. *Ibid.*

19. Sandison, Whitelaw, Spencer. *Op. Cit.*

20. Robert de Ropp. *Drugs and the Mind*, 236 ff.

21. Sandison, Whitelaw, Spencer. *Op. Cit.*

22. *Ibid.*

23. Sandison and Whitelaw. *Op. Cit.*

24. Sandison. "The Clinical Uses of LSD."

25. Walter Frederking. "Intoxicant Drugs (LSD and Mecaline) in Psychotherapy." *Journal of Nervous and Mental Diseases*. Vol. 121. Pp. 262 ff.

26. Cholden, Albert Kurland, Charles Savage. "Clinical Reactions and Tolerances to LSD in Chronic Schizophrenia." *Journal of Nervous and Mental Diseases*. Vol. 122. Pp. 211 ff.

27. Betty Eisner and Sidney Cohen. "Psychotherapy with LSD." *Journal of Nervous and Mental Diseases*. Vol. 127. Pp. 525 ff.

28. Ian Stevenson. "Comments on the Psychological Effects of Mescaline and Allied Drugs." *Journal of Nervous and Mental Diseases*. Vol. 125. Pp. 438 ff.

29. Sandison. *Op. Cit.*

APPENDIX B

1. *Collected Papers*. Vol. I. Pp. 148 ff.

2. P. 150.

3. *The Origins of Psychoanalysis*, 218 ff. Italics mine.

4. *Collected Papers*. Vol. I. P. 215.

5. *The Basic Writings*, 940. Italics mine.

6. *Introductory Lectures on Psychoanalysis*, 307 ff.

7. *An Autobiographical Study*, 62 ff. Italics mine.

APPENDIX C

1. Breuer and Freud. *Studies on Hysteria*, 202.

2. Freud. *The Interpretation of Dreams*, 178.

3. Neal E. Miller. "Theory and Experiment Relating Psychoanalytic Displacement to Stimulus Response Generalization." *Journal of Abnormal and Social Psychology*. Vol. 43. Pp. 155 ff.

4. *On Dreams*, 15.

5. Freud. *Totem and Taboo*, 129.

6. Freud. *Collected Papers*. Vol. II. P. 64.

APPENDIX D

1. *Introductory Lectures on Psychoanalysis*, 145. Italics mine.
2. *Basic Writings*, 647.
3. P. 642.
4. *Ibid.*
5. P. 652.
6. *The Interpretation of Dreams*, 383.
7. *Introductory Lectures*, 98, 99.
8. *Interpretation of Dreams*, 427 ff.

APPENDIX E

1. *The Origins of Psychoanalysis*, 157.
2. *Collected Papers.* Vol. I. P. 159.
3. *The Interpretation of Dreams*, 418.
4. *Ibid.* Italics mine.
5. *Collected Papers.* Vol. I. P. 37.
6. *New Introductory Lectures on Psychoanalysis*, 200 ff.
7. *An Outline of Psychoanalysis*, 83 ff.
8. P. 84.

BIBLIOGRAPHY

Abramson, Harold: "LSD as an Adjunct to Psychotherapy with Elimination of the Fear of Homosexuality." *Journal of Psychology.* Vol. 39. 1955.

———: "LSD as an Adjunct to Brief Psychotherapy with Special Reference to Ego Enhancement." *Journal of Psychology.* Vol. 41. 1956.

———, ed.: "The Use of LSD in Psychotherapy." Josiah H. Macy Foundation. 1960.

———, M. P. Hewitt, H. Lennard, W. J. Turner, F. J. O'Neill, S. Merlis: "The Stablemate Concept of Therapy as Affected by LSD in Schizophrenia." *Journal of Psychology.* Vol. 45. 1958.

Bercel, Nicholas, Lee Travis, Leonard Olinger, Erik Dreikurs: "Model Psychosis Induced by LSD in Normals." *Archives of Neurology and Psychiatry.* Vol. 75. 1956.

Bockoven, J. Sanbourne: "Explorations in Psychotherapy." *Archives of Neurology and Psychiatry.* Vol. 80. 1958.

Breuer, Joseph, and Sigmund Freud: *Studies on Hysteria.* London. Hogarth. 1956.

Busch, Anthony K., and Warren C. Johnson: "LSD as an Aid to Psychotherapy." *Diseases of the Nervous System.* Vol. 11. 1950.

Chandler, Arthur, and Mortimer Hartman: "LSD as a Facilitating Agent in Psychotherapy." *Archives of Neurology and Psychiatry.* January 1960.

Cholden, Louis, Albert Kurland, and Charles Savage: "Clinical Reactions and Tolerances to LSD in Chronic Schizophrenia." *Journal of Nervous and Mental Diseases.* Vol. 122. 1955.

Cholden, Louis, ed.: *LSD and Mescaline in Experimental Psychiatry.* New York. Grune and Stratton. 1956.

De Ropp, Robert: *Drugs and the Mind.* New York. St. Martin's Press. 1957.

Eisner, Betty, and Sidney Cohen: "Psychotherapy with LSD." *Journal of Nervous and Mental Diseases.* Vol. 127. 1958.

Encyclopaedia Britannica. New York. 1958.

English, O. Spurgeon, and Gerald Pearson: *Emotional Problems of Living.* New York. Norton. 1955.

Frederking, Walter: "Intoxicant Drugs (LSD and Mescaline) in Psychotherapy." *Journal of Nervous and Mental Diseases.* Vol. 121. 1955.

Freud, Sigmund: *An Autobiographical Study.* New York. Norton. 1952.

———: *Basic Writings.* New York. Modern Library. 1938.

Freud, Sigmund: *Collected Papers.* Vol. I-V. London. Hogarth. 1956.

———: *The Ego and the Id.* London. Hogarth. 1957.

———: *The Interpretation of Dreams.* London. Allen and Unwin. 1951.

———: *Introductory Lectures on Psychoanalysis.* London. Allen and Unwin. 1952.

———: *Leonardo da Vinci.* London. Routledge and Kegan Paul. 1948.

———: *New Introductory Lectures on Psychoanalysis.* New York. Norton. 1933.

———: *On Dreams.* London. Hogarth. 1952.

———: *Origins of Psychoanalysis.* New York. Doubleday Anchor. 1957.

———: *An Outline of Psychoanalysis.* New York. Norton. 1949.

———: *The Question of Lay Analysis.* New York. Norton. 1950.

———: *Totem and Taboo.* London. Routledge *et al.* 1950.

Funk and Wagnall: *College Standard Dictionary.* New York. 1937.

Giberti, F., and G. Boeri: "Studio Farmacopsichiatrico di un Caso di Nevrosi Fobico-Ansiosa." *Sistema Nervoso.* Vol. 9. 1957.

Garattini and Ghetti, eds.: *Psychotropic Drugs.* New York. Elsevier. 1957.

Hoch, Paul: "Remarks on LSD and Mescaline." *Journal of Nervous and Mental Diseases.* Vol. 122. 1957.

Hoffer, Abram, Humphrey Osmond, and John Smythies: "Schizophrenia, A New Approach." *Journal of Mental Science.* Vol. 100. 1954.

Hoffer, Abram, and Humphrey Osmond: "The Adrenochrome Model and Schizophrenia." *Journal of Nervous and Mental Diseases.* Vol. 128. 1959.

Huxley, Aldous: *Heaven and Hell.* New York. Harper. 1956.

———: "Drugs That Shape Men's Minds." *Saturday Evening Post.* October 1958.

Janiger, Oscar: "The Use of Hallucinogenic Agents in Psychiatry." *California Clinician.* July–August 1959.

Jost, F. "Zur therapeutischen Verwendung des LSD-25 in der Klinischen Praxis der Psychiatrie." *Wiener Klinische Wochenschrift.* Vol. 69. 1957.

Jung, Carl: *Practice of Psychotherapy.* New York. Bollingen. 1954.

———: *The Archetypes and the Collective unconscious.* New York. Bollingen. 1959.

———: *Voice of America Broadcast.* 1956.

Kety, Seymour, ed.: "Pharmacology of Psychotomimetic and Psychotherapeutic Drugs." *Annals of New York Academy of Science.* Vol. 66. 1957.

Kinsey, Alfred, Wendell Pomeroy, Clyde Martin, and Paul Gebhard: *Sexual Behavior in the Human Female.* Philadelphia. Saunders. 1953.

Kornetsky, Conan: "Relation of Physiological and Psychological Effects of LSD." *Archives of Neurology and Psychiatry.* Vol. 77. 1959.

Lewis, Sloane: "Therapy with LSD." *Journal of Clinical and Experimental Psychopathology.* Vol. 19. 1958.

Los Angeles Times. March 27, 1960.

Martin, A. Joyce: "LSD Treatment of Chronic Psychoneurotics Under Day Hospital Conditions." *International Journal of Social Psychiatry*. Vol. 3. 1957.

Miller, Neal E.: "Theory and Experiment Relating Psychoanalytic Displacement to Stimulus Response Generalization." *Journal of Abnormal and Social Psychology*. Vol. 143. 1948.

Pavlov, Ivan: *Conditioned Reflexes*. London. Oxford University Press. 1927.

Pennes, Harry: "Clinical Experiences with New Hallucinogens." *Annals of New York Academy of Science*. Ed. Kety. Vol. 66. 1957.

———, editor: Psychopharmacology: *Pharmacological Effects of Behavior*. New York. Hoeber-Harper. 1958.

Rinkel, Max, and Herman C. Denber, eds.: *Chemical Concepts of Psychosis*. New York. McDowell, Obolensky. 1958.

Rinkel, Max, and Harry Solomon: "Experimental Psychiatry: A Chemical Concept of Psychosis." *Diseases of the Nervous System*. Vol. 15. 1954.

Rinkel, Max. "Pharmacodynamics of LSD and Mescaline." *Journal of Nervous and Mental Diseases*. Vol. 125. 1957.

Rothlin, Ernst. "Pharmacology of LSD." *LSD and Mescaline in Experimental Psychiatry*. Cf. Cholden.

———: "Pharmacology of LSD and Some of Its Related Compounds." *Psychotropic Drugs*. Eds. Garattini and Ghetti. New York. Elsevier. 1957.

Sandison, Ronald, J. D. A. Whitelaw, and A. M. Spencer: "Therapeutic Value of LSD in Mental Illness." *Journal of Mental Science*. Vol. 100. 1957.

Sandison, Ronald, and J. D. A. Whitelaw: "Further Studies in the Therapeutic Value of LSD in Mental Illness." *Journal of Mental Science*. Vol. 103. 1957.

Sandison, Ronald. "Clinical Uses of LSD." In *LSD and Mescaline in Experimental Psychiatry*. Cf. Cholden.

Savage, Charles. "LSD, A Clinical-Psychological Study." *Americal Journal of Psychiatry*. Vol. 108. 1952.

———: "Variations of Ego Feelings Induced by LSD." *Psychoanalytic Revue*. Vol. 42. 1955.

———: "Resolution and Subsequent Remobilization of Resistance by LSD in Psychotherapy." *Journal of Nervous and Mental Diseases*. Vol. 125. 1957.

———, and Louis Cholden: "Schizophrenia and the Model Psychosis." *Journal of Clinical and Experimental Psychopathology*. Vol. 17. 1956.

Schwartz, Bert, Carl Sem-Jacobson, and Magnus Peterson: "Effects of LSD, Mescaline, and Adrenoxine on Depth Electrograms in Man." *Archives of Neurology and Psychiatry*. Vol. 75. 1956.

Stevenson, Ian. "Comments on the Psychological Effects of Mescaline and Allied Drugs." *Journal of Nervous and Mental Diseases*. Vol. 125. 1957.

Stoll, W. A. "Lysergsaure diathylamid, ein Phantastikum aus der Mutterkorngruppe." *Schweizerland Archives fon Neurologie und Psychiatrie*. Vol. 60. 1947.

Terrell, Paul. "I Went Experimentally Insane" (as told to Ted Levine). *Argosy*. August 1959.

Toledo, Fontana, Morales: "Psychoanalysis and LSD: Basis for a Combined Technique." *Acta Neuropsychiatria.* Vol. 4. 1958.

Tors, Ivan. *Impressions Received After Taking LSD.* 1959. Unpublished.

Watson, John B., and Rosalie Reyner: "Conditioned Emotional Reactions." *Journal of Experimental Psychology.* Vol. 3. 1920.

Wikler, Abraham: *Relation of Psychiatry to Pharmacology.* Baltimore. Waverly. 1957.

Wolfe, Thomas. *Look Homeward, Angel.* New York. Scribner's. 1929.

Some may close their eyes to Mrs. Newland's shattering revelations by dismissing her as disturbed or sick. If so, it will be only because they are not ready to bring her kind of courage to the task of self-inspection. For this is not the account of the struggle of a schizophrenic or a crippled neurotic, but the further advance to self-realization of an already efficient, able member of society.

With excitement we follow the author's sometimes terrifying, sometimes amusing journey through inexplicable nightmares and weird fantasies. We see the intricate, fascinating process by which patient and therapist unlock the unconscious and purge the depths of human neg-

ativity. The whole baffling problem of frigidity in the liberally educated woman—who consciously has accepted her right to sexual pleasure but whose unconscious holds her frozen in the grip of destroying terrors and rages—is explored with unprecedented candor. The complex fabric of early relationships and experiences—rather than conscious anti-sexual teachings—is revealed as the pleasure-destroying element. *"The intimate explorations of a woman's sexual life by a woman is practically unique in literature,"* Dr. Harold Greenwald writes in the foreword to MY SELF AND I. *"Most such accounts have been perceptive and intuitive but none has been able to tell us so much about the inner experiences of a woman's sexual response."*

CONSTANCE A. NEWLAND, the pseudonym for the author of MY SELF AND I, describes herself as a housewife with two children whom she cares for by pursuing a career as a writer. Formerly a stage and screen actress, she has published a novel and written for Broadway, television and

motion pictures. Her life is filled with the social and professional rewards of a gifted, attractive woman.

JACKET DESIGN BY BEN FEDER, INC.

Coward-McCann, Inc.
200 Madison Avenue
New York 16, N. Y.